Marketing for The Legal Nurse Consultant

A guide to getting all the clients you can handle using proven, low cost strategies

Betty Joos, R.N., B.S.N., M.Ed, LNC
John Joos, M.B.A., D.B.A.

Sky Lake Publishing
www.sky-lake.com

100 Falling Creek
Sautee, GA 30571

888-SKY-LAKE
Sky Lake Publishing
P. O. Box 219
Sautee, Georgia 30571
skylakepub@sky-lake.com

PUBLISHER CATALOGING-IN-PUBLICATION DATA

Joos, Betty & Joos, John

Marketing for the Legal Nurse Consultant: A guide to getting all the clients you can handle using proven, low cost strategies.

Includes index and bibliographic references.
ISBN 0-9674730-0-4
1. Legal Nurse Consultant. 2. Marketing. 3. Marketing-costs.

Library of Congress Catalog Card Number: **99-91290**

Contents At A Glance

Table of Contents

A note from the Authors:

Dr. John

I'm not a nurse, but I sleep with one. I call her "Nurse Betty." She is the light of my life and a true soul mate.

We decided to write this book because of the many discussions we have had with nurses who called our video production company, Sky Lake Productions, to order our Legal Nurse Consultant Profiles video and other LNC resources. It didn't take us long to realize that many of our nurse-clients wanted, and needed, information about how to market their practice. This book is an opportunity to apply what I teach to graduate students in Masters of Business Administration marketing and customer service courses at Nova Southeastern University. It also is an opportunity to share many of the lessons I have learned from the clients of my small business consulting practice and our video production company.

As a concession to Nurse Betty, I have agreed to label all my comments with the heading, "John Sez." I believe she thinks my humor is a bit "out there" at times. The nurse decided to label hers with "Betty's comments."

We had a great time writing this book. And our marriage is still intact despite our many discussions about the content, form, and format of this book. I am particularly proud of the fact that during the writing of this book I never heard the words "doofus" or "are you completely crazy" escape from Nurse Betty's mouth.

John Joos, B.S., M.B.A., D.B.A.

A note from the Authors (Continued):

Nurse Betty

Well, I am a nurse and have been a legal nurse consultant since 1988 (even before we had an organization that named us "legal nurse consultants"). My experience began with working in a defense law firm before I went out "on my own" as an independent LNC. Thus, my contribution to this labor of love is from my own experiences in the world of legal "goings-on."

I have maintained, and grown, an independent practice for a decade. I have also been involved in developing curriculum for LNCs and have taught medical research and writing as well as marketing to future LNCs. Therefore, what we have here is a good mix of personal experience and academic knowledge (his as well as mine).

One last statement relating to this book: If you have not yet informed yourself thoroughly about what a legal nurse consultant does and how to do it, you are not yet ready for this book. This marketing book assumes you already have the preparation for becoming a legal nurse consultant – otherwise, you do not know what your "product" is.

Betty Joos, R.N., B.S.N., M.Ed., LNC

Acknowledgements

We have had good tips and bad experiences related to us from friends in this business. We have learned a great deal from friends like Jenny Beerman, Peggy Camp, Agnes Grogan, Pat Steed, Claudette Varanko, Marlene Vermeer-Campbell, and Paula Woo, independent LNCs who participated in our Profiles video. Other successful LNCs have also provided helpful insights. In teaching marketing to future LNCs in the Atlanta area, I learned even more about the process of marketing and have learned from some of my students as well. Nadine Neville-Turpin, a former student, has shown herself to be an outstanding marketer. She and Leslie Hardison Knicely, another successful LNC, read the drafts for us and provided valuable input. Carin Gordon, an attorney and educator, also read manuscript drafts and offered her knowledge and encouragement in this venture. Our thanks go to all those who have offered encouragement and interest in the project and gave us additional ideas.

We have referred often to the professional organization, The American Association of Legal Nurse Consultants and highly recommend that any nurse who plans to do this work should join AALNC. Both the local and national associations have a great deal to offer in guidance, education, and networking. Our thanks to all members, past and present, who make this organization so worthwhile.

> To love what you do and feel that it matters – how could anything be
> more fun?
> *Katherine Graham*

SECTION I – INTRODUCTION

Marketing is everything you do to promote your business. Letters, brochures, calls, networking, free publicity, testimonials, talks, recommendations, referrals, and writing articles are examples of the wide variety of marketing tools available to the Legal Nurse Consultant. You could say that "marketing is a state of mind." You should consider anyone you meet a potential source of new clients.

BEFORE YOU START

Learning about marketing yourself assumes you have prepared for the business service you offer. Are you prepared? If you cannot respond positively to the following list of items, you have more work to do before you start your active marketing.

1. Are you informed about what you as an LNC can specifically do for a client? If not:
    - ❑ Take a study course specifically for LNCs
    - ❑ Prepare independently with guidance from other LNCs
    - ❑ Learn from AALNC members/organizations

2. Do you have the ability to provide clients with professionally done reports? You must:
    ☐ Have a computer with a good word-processing program and know how to use it.
    ☐ Have a computer with a connection to the Internet and know how to do medical literature research as well as locate other information as needed.
    ☐ Have the skills and ability to prepare well-written, thoroughly edited, time-saving, and informative work product for your clients.
    ☐ If no computer, have a dictating machine and a word-processing professional whom you can subcontract.

3. Do you have office supplies and dedicated office space to use for business purposes? You should:
    ☐ Have a separate, protected space in which you can do your work without fear of losing or damaging the medical records or without compromising confidentiality of the records or your report.
    ☐ Have safe filing containers (can be as simple as sturdy boxes) to store records/reports when you are not working on them.
    ☐ Have a laser printer (preferable) or at least a good quality ink jet printer for reports and correspondence.
    ☐ Have a separate phone line or at least an identifiable ring on your home line for your business use.
    ☐ Have office supplies such as file folders, sticky notes, shipping supplies (check out the available shipping containers at the post office), paper clips (all sizes

and types), slip sheets, staple machine, staple remover, stationery, etc.

4. Do you have a plan for your fee structure, billing process, and client information? You need to:
   ❑ Know what your fees will be before you start marketing.
   ❑ Have a form for specific and consistent client information.
   ❑ Know your format for billing hours and preparing invoices.

5. Do you have your stationery, business cards, brochures, resume, etc. prepared?
   ❑ This book will help you plan those for the most impact, but they should be ready before you start your active marketing.

6. Have you consulted with your family and discussed how this new business may affect all of them?
   ❑ Your spouse should not only be agreeable to the new business but should also be supportive.
   ❑ Your children, according their ability (by age) to understand, should be included in the discussion.
   ❑ Be certain you have the time to take on this extra work if you plan to continue your current position.

You must be able to respond positively to almost all these points before you start marketing yourself actively—meaning before you start mailing out materials or calling/contacting clients. This book offers help on some items—such as developing brochures, business cards, and other marketing materials. However, you must have the skills and knowledge as well as the specific equipment to be prepared to provide this service to law firms, insurance companies, etc. This book does not purport to teach you <u>how</u> to be a legal nurse consultant; it offers ways to help you find, get, and keep clients for those skills you bring.

With that understood, lets get started.

THE MISTAKE MADE BY MANY NURSES GOING INTO BUSINESS

It is a mistake to assume that, because you have many years of nursing experience and offer excellent services, new prospects for your legal nurse consulting career will automatically seek

Your mission is to let everyone who needs your services know about them....

you out for your services. This rarely happens. In the beginning, you must proactively build a client base by aggressively marketing yourself and your services. To do otherwise smacks of either arrogance, if not stupidity (do we have your attention yet?).

Your mission is to let everyone who needs your services know about them and to do so in a way that convinces them to contact YOU when they have such a need. Professional marketers call this needs-based marketing.

Many nurses who are going into business never understand the concept of needs-based marketing. More often than not, jobs in the nursing profession have simply required that you show up with a valid state nursing license for a job interview. Your license is accepted as proof of both your education and your "expertise." LNCs also need a valid nursing license, but your nursing license does not, in this case, indicate any expertise in the medical-legal arena.

WHAT EVERY LNC MUST SELL

As an independent LNC, you will be selling your knowledge and expertise to clients who may not have a good appreciation of what you can do for them. They do not necessarily care about your long list of CEUs or your latest performance appraisal as a nurse. They do care about their needs. They want to know what you can do for them, how soon you can do it, and at what cost. Of course, this is predicated on the fact that YOU know what you can do for the client and can impress that client with the value of your services.

In order to be successful as a Legal Nurse Consultant, you must sell the potential client (the attorney, insurance company, state agency, etc.) on your total package. This includes professional looking marketing materials, your professional appearance and behavior, and your excellent work product. That is what this marketing guide sets out to do - to help you present yourself and your services in the best possible way to potential clients. We assume you already have knowledge of how legal nurse consulting is done.

...to be successful as a Legal Nurse Consultant, you must sell the potential client... on your total package.

STEAL SHAMELESSLY FROM THIS GUIDE

All of our guide materials are copyrighted. However, as a purchaser of the guide, you are authorized to adapt any examples of letters, brochures, or other marketing materials included in the guide for your own personal use in marketing your practice. On the other hand, you are not authorized to use this material to create materials for re-sale to others - as in developing your own marketing book or materials for sale.

The only advice we offer is that you change the wording of the examples in order to save the embarrassment of sending the same material to a potential client that other LNCs who have used this guide may send.

A NOTE ON CERTIFICATION

We hear from many nurses interested in doing legal nurse consulting and a common question is, "Is certification required?" The answer is that you are not required to be certified to do legal nurse consulting. Like most other fields of specialty nursing, certification usually indicates that you have developed an expertise in that field.

...you are not required to be certified to do legal nurse consulting

The American Association of Legal Nurse Consultants offers a certification for those who can pass the AALNC's exam and show evidence of a specific amount of experience in the field of legal nurse consulting. In accordance with the ANA certification recommendations, a BS will be a certification requirement as well. You can do LNC work without being certified. Certification is a more a "nurse thing" than an "attorney thing." Most attorneys are more interested in what you can do for them and how soon you can do it. Of course, you are certainly more likely to do a better job with experience as well as training in the field. With or without certification, your job is to provide an exceptional work product in the way of thoroughness, neatness, unbiased, and well-researched correct information from the outset of your consulting career.

Certification is more a "nurse thing" than an "attorney thing."

Betty's comment:
As more LNCs become certified by the AALNC, it is likely that certification will become an additional marketing tool. However, it will never be a substitute for good, basic marketing skills.

Further information on certification can be obtained from:

American Association of Legal Nurse Consultants

4700 West Lake Avenue,

Glenview, IL 60025-1485

877-402-2562

WWW.AALNC.ORG

The Bottom Line

☑ Before your start, be prepared.

☑ To be successful you must actively seek business.

☑ You must sell clients on the total package that includes you, your expertise, and your ability to solve their problems.

☑ Certification, while a plus, is not required.

☑ The resources provided in this book are available for your personal use. Steal all that are useful.

My greatest strength as a consultant is to be ignorant
and to ask a few questions.
Peter Drucker

SECTION 2 – NEEDS-BASED MARKETING

In this section you will learn about needs-based marketing. It is a simple and powerful concept of helping your clients meet their needs related to medical-legal issues. Understanding needs-based marketing will put you miles ahead of your competition.

THE DIFFERENCE BETWEEN THE SELLING APPROACH AND THE NEEDS-BASED APPROACH

When you think of yourself as a Legal Nurse Consultant who helps clients solve their problems, your whole approach to marketing changes. You are then no longer just another nurse trying to sell your services; instead, you're a consultant who is always looking for prospects with problems and thinking of ways you can use your knowledge, skills, and abilities to develop solutions to those problems. Not much different from clinical nursing, is it?

...you are a resource to your client instead of someone who is selling something.

> **John Sez:**
> By both training and inclination, nursing is a profession that is skilled at understanding and meeting a patient's needs. Therefore, "needs-based marketing" is a logical extension of a skill set that many nurses already have. You may be surprised to discover that needs-based marketing is a lot like nursing except there are no bedpans involved in the process.

In many instances, you will be dealing with prospective clients who may have never given a thought to using the services of a Legal Nurse Consultant or may not know what an LNC is. This will require you to educate the attorney about your services as well as provide consulting on a case. Clients may recognize the need related to medical issues but are unaware that you are able to help solve their specific problems. In other instances, clients and prospects will recognize you as a consultant who is the source of helpful information regarding their specific medical case issues. What you must get across is that you are a resource to your client instead of someone who is selling something.

Who is your client?

The LNC does NOT work for the actual named plaintiff[s] or defendant[s] but is contracted (as an independent) to provide a service for the attorneys who represent these clients. Additionally, LNCs may provide services for insurance companies, state or federal agencies, hospitals, or other agencies that deal with medical-legal issues. Understanding who your clients are helps you to focus on what their needs are or may be.

Understanding who your clients are helps you to focus on what their needs are...

Your clients need help to solve their problems

Your job then is to position yourself as a problem solver rather than a seller of services. You have answers, or can find them through research, to the client's need for medical information,

ou have the answers...or can find them....

explanation, summarization, interpretation, or other medical/ nursing expertise.

Your goals should be: (1) to present yourself as confident in your abilities to help solve problems related to medical-legal issues; and (2) to educate the client as to what you can do to help them present the best possible strategy in cases with medical-legal issues.

John Sez:

Don't underestimate the "Embarrassment Factor"(I call it the "EF").
Many people are motivated to behaviors that are calculated to avoid embarrassment. Attorneys are no different. They want to win cases. Losing cases, or even being in error about medical points of the case, can be a big EF. LNCs who understand this do what they can to help their clients avoid the EF.

WHAT YOUR PROSPECTS AND CLIENTS ARE *REALLY* INTERESTED IN

Your clients are interested in winning cases, competently

Your clients are interested in winning cases...

representing their clients, and not being caught off-guard or being embarrassed by the opposing side.

These are some of the problems that concern your prospects. Clients and prospects will pay attention to people who can help

LNCs position themselves as problem-solvers and consultants...

them solve their problems. This is why successful LNCs position themselves as problem-solvers and consultants who offer

benefits and solutions to their clients.

Clients' and prospects' needs encompass not only medical records review and analysis but also information on how the hospital/doctors' office/HMO systems work. They may have a need to be educated on specific medical topics for which you can provide authoritative research. They may need to locate and obtain a medical expert – after you help them determine what type of expert would be best for their current case. They may need help in preparing for medical depositions. State and Federal agencies may need help in identifying fraudulent care or billing. Hospitals may need help in identifying potential litigation issues prior to a lawsuit occurrence as well as after the fact (risk management issues).

Needs-based marketing requires that you know your client well enough to understand their specific needs. In the case of a client who has little experience working with LNCs, you also may have to take the time to help the client identify and understand their needs. Once both of you have a common understanding of the needs, you are in a position to offer benefits and solutions.

The Good News

The good news is that attorneys have traditionally used a needs-based approach to market their own services. Until recent years, Bar Association rules prevented attorneys from advertising their services. Consequently, most law firms developed a marketing approach that centered on trying to understand potential clients' needs and convincing the client that the firm/attorney could meet those needs. A needs-based approach fits with the legal industry quite well. This same approach also works when marketing to insurance companies or hospital risk management departments.

THE 80/20 RULE OF COMMUNICATION

When communicating with a client in any manner, **eighty percent** or more of the content

...eighty percent or more of the content should be about the client

should be about the client, their problems, and what you can do to help. **Twenty percent** or less should be about you and even that should be geared to reinforcing the knowledge, skills, and abilities that you can bring to solve the problems presented by the medical issues. The 80/20 rule applies to all of your marketing materials as well.

John Sez:
Here's how this works:: Listen, listen, listen, listen, talk, listen, listen, listen...

The Bottom Line

☑ Successful LNCs think of themselves as problem solvers rather then someone who is "selling something."

☑ You and your clients must have a common agreement of what the "needs" are.

☑ Don't overlook the "Embarrassment Factor."

☑ Clients will listen to someone who they feel understands their problems and who can offer solutions.

☑ 80% of your communication should be "client-focused."

☑ Listen aggressively.

When one door closes, another opens. But we so often look so long
and so regretfully upon the closed door that we do not see the one
which has been opened for us.
Alexander Graham Bell

SECTION 3 - FINDING YOUR NICHE

This section will help you understand the importance of setting
yourself apart by having a niche. You will learn the difference
between an LNC and a nurse expert witness and the difference
between an LNC and a "nurse-paralegal."

FIND YOUR NICHE

Many new LNCs start out taking any case work that comes in
the door, whether it is plaintiff or defense, medical malpractice,
personal injury, workers' compensation, or another medically
related case. That may work for a while, but to market yourself
well, it helps to pick a niche, or focus, for your work. Maybe
you prefer plaintiff work to defense work—or vice-versa. Maybe
you have exceptional research skills you want to emphasize.
Maybe you prefer doing personal injury, or workers'
compensation, or medical malpractice, or forensic cases, or
products liability, or health law issues, or nursing home cases,
or risk management. You get the picture.

> John Sez:
> Nursing Home and Assisted Living cases are a hot growth area in the legal field. As the baby boom generation begins to retire, elder care cases are springing up like mushrooms after a hard rain.
> If you have nursing home or assisted living expertise, you may become a hot commodity in the LNC marketplace.

There are many choices that you can make. You can offer your services as someone with advanced knowledge and skills in the area of your niche. Becoming somewhat specialized will often

Being a "specialist" … means you will emphasize a specific area of legal issues

get you more work than being a generalist. As a behind-the-scenes consultant, you will still provide services for all types of medical issues even if you have a niche focus. Being a "specialist" does not mean you would only do orthopedic cases or emergency room cases; it means you will emphasize a specific area of legal issues rather than medical issues. (Although we are beginning to see a few LNCs who are building a good practice by just doing obstetric cases or nursing home cases, etc.—it is still the exception rather than the rule.)

> John Sez:
> Don't get all carried away with this niche thing. Many successful LNCs limit themselves to either plaintiff or defense for the majority of their cases. Niches are developed as LNCs get a foothold in the marketplace. The current state of things is that most LNCs have to combine several niches in order to produce a viable income stream. (Can you say "positive cash flow?")

If your niche is researching and writing reports of the medical-legal issues—you can market yourself as a specialist to other LNCs as well as to law firms, health agencies, government groups, or risk management. This is particularly effective when you are skilled at online research as well as library research—in fact, you must be skilled at Internet searching to specialize in research and writing.

If you have had experience doing workers' compensation cases, which have very specialized state-controlled rules and regulations, you have a distinct advantage over someone who does not know those requirements.

Deciding between specializing in plaintiff work or defense work certainly makes it easier to avoid a conflict of interest (covered later in this section) when choosing or accepting clients. On the other hand, in order to have a sufficient volume of work, you may have to seek clients in several niches. Medical malpractice and products liability cases seem to fit well together. Doing all defense work or all plaintiff work is also a choice if you <u>don't</u> do expert witness work. (See the discussion about nurse expert witnesses following.)

,... in order to have a sufficient volume of work, you may have to seek clients in several niches.

Medical Malpractice cases are not the only cases LNCs consult on

Many LNCs, as well as attorneys, think of using a nurse-consultant only in med mal cases. This can limit your ability to generate income. There are also products liability cases related to drugs or devices; personal injury cases which usually involve no medical standard of care but do involve injury issues; workers' compensation cases which may be short lived but make up for that in sheer numbers of cases. An LNC might contract risk-management work in small hospitals. Don't limit your choice of possible niches in a way that prevents you from having enough business. However, do have a focus.

The three things you need to determine your niche

Three things you need to help in determining your niche are the available time to work as an LNC, your medical-legal experience, and a sense of the available market for your choice. When starting out as an LNC, you may not have enough information to make such a decision. If you start out a generalist, meaning you do all types of cases for both plaintiff and defense, you will eventually become aware of what type of case work you do well—and like. You will also develop a sense of whether there is sufficient market to support your niche choice.

...you may not have enough information to make.... a decision

As the number of attorneys using LNCs grows and there is more competition in the marketplace, you may have the opportunity to differentiate yourself through some very specific niche skills and knowledge such as only doing nursing home/geriatric cases. Currently that is not always the case.

Betty's comment:
Attorneys frequently specialize, though some solo practice attorneys also take "all cases coming through the door." Most attorneys have an area of specialty such as family law, personal injury, etc. It isn't that they won't take any other type of case, but, ethically, they are not always able to offer the best representation outside their area of expertise.

LNCs AS COMPARED TO NURSE EXPERT WITNESSES

Legal Nurse Consultants' work referred to above is "behind-the-scenes" consulting—not expert witness work. Table 3-1, located at the end of section 3, lists examples of behind-the-scenes consulting. (Hint - Some of the items in table 3-1 may be worth stealing for use as brochure or cover letter language.)

Nurse expert witnesses may perform many of the same services listed in Table 3-1. However, when you position yourself as a nurse expert witness, <u>it is in the context of a nursing issue only.</u>

The nurse expert witness, to be most effective, should have current clinical nursing expertise in the area under litigation. This can be somewhat limiting in the type of case on which the nurse can effectively work. The nurse expert witness can expect to be deposed by the side opposite from which she is hired as the expert. The integrity and background of the nurse are "fair game" for denigrating by the other side. They will want to minimize the effect the nurse's testimony will have. It may also require going to trial to present testimony. Both these situations—deposition and trial—can be great stress-producers. If you have any type of stage fright, this may not be a good choice of niche for you.

> **Betty's comment:**
> As a nurse expert, you need to do both plaintiff and defense cases to avoid even the appearance of bias in your opinions towards one side or the other. A question often asked of testifying experts is how many of each —plaintiff or defense— have you done.

Another big problem with being positioned as an expert witness is that, unlike a behind-the-scenes consultant, all of your "work product," i.e., notes, letters, communications, reports, etc., will be "discoverable" by the other side. Discoverable means that the other side is allowed access to them (they may get copies of everything you write, including scrap paper notes, letters, e-mail). In some situations, experts may be asked by the hiring attorney not to make any written notes regarding the

Another big problem… is that… all of your "work product," …will be "discoverable" by the other side.

case until they are asked to do so. This is not the situation with the work done by the LNC acting behind-the-scenes—their "work product" is almost always a written report and is not discoverable (except under very occasional and specific circumstances).

There are attorneys who think that LNCs are used only as expert witnesses in nursing malpractice cases. This misconception limits the possibility that an attorney will think about using your services as a behind-the-scene consultant in other situations. This is why educating potential clients about the full range of what you can do for them is so important.

WHY THERE ARE "SLIM PICKINGS" FOR NURSE EXPERT WITNESSES

Most medical malpractice cases are not against nurses, and thus a nurse who only does expert witness work may find cases few *Many nurse expert witnesses have a history of having researched and published...* and far between. You also must have expertise in the nursing issues being litigated. Many nurse expert witnesses have a history of having researched and published in their area of expertise. This makes them more valuable–if their research supports the issue being litigated.

John Sez:
As an expert witness you will be subject to having your testimony challenged by the opposing attorneys. This can be brutal. Especially since they don't administer anesthesia. "Losing it" on the witness stand is not a big plus.

Marketing done by medical or nursing experts must be done with exceptional care in order to prevent the appearance of being a "hired gun." A "hired gun" is an expert who is seen as hired only to agree with what the attorneys want you to say. You must be careful to protect your integrity from this potential label.

Being a nurse expert witness is a niche market in itself. It can be highly lucrative work. Expert

Being a nurse expert witness... can be highly lucrative work.

witnesses charge a higher rate per hour than behind-the-scenes consultants. Giving depositions and going to trial in a case can be a greater stress-producer than just reviewing and writing reports. This fact is reflected in a higher hourly fee at deposition and, often, an even higher hourly fee in court. Remember also that, as the "expert," the "buck stops with you." If a nurse expert witness has published anything on the topic being litigated or has been used as an expert on the same topic in other cases, you can be sure the testimony given in deposition and trial will be compared with previous testimony or publications. You should also be aware that the "other side" will likely have a nurse expert as well. And their expert may present the issues in a different light than you.

DOING BOTH BEHIND-THE-SCENES AND EXPERT WITNESS WORK

It is possible to do both types of LNC work—as an expert in your field of expertise and as a behind-the-scene consultant. When doing behind-the-scenes consulting, you may likely be reviewing records from cases that do not involve your clinical specialty. It is occasionally difficult to get the attorney to see you as able to provide support in both ways. This requires further education of your attorney-client but can be a good way to extend the client relationship.

THE DIFFERENCE BETWEEN AN LNC AND A "NURSE-PARALEGAL"

In the early days of legal nurse consulting, some nurses became paralegals in order to get their foot in the door with attorneys. Nurses were not recognized for their role as consultants since they were often called "nurse-paralegals" and functioned in the role as a specialized paralegal—not as a nurse with specific medical-as-well-as-nursing expertise. In 1989, the American Association of Legal Nurse Consultants (AALNC) came into being and began to position the LNC as a nursing specialty. Here's the big difference; independent LNCs charge from around $50 per hour to above $120 per hour for their services. Paralegals, as a rule, are paid significantly less. An LNC who sails under the banner of nurse-paralegal often will be thought of as a paralegal who has "some" medical expertise and is likely to be paid accordingly.

John Sez:
Q: What's the difference between a paralegal and an LNC?
Ans: About $60 per hour.

A contextual difference between the nurse-paralegal and the LNC is that the nurse-paralegal is often used as a paralegal without reference to specialized skills and knowledge that comes with a nursing background. The AALNC has published a Position Statement (JLNC, Apr 1999, Vol 10(2); 33) defining legal nurse consulting as a specialty practice of nursing – not as a special category of paralegals. LNCs are consulted "because of their expertise in nursing and health care." For this reason, and for good business reasons, LNCs have been trying to put some distance between themselves and paralegals. Remember, it was only a century ago that barbers and doctors were considered the same profession. You are aware that doctors have put a great distance between themselves and barbers? Think about it.

CONFLICT OF INTEREST

Conflict of interest, or the perception of such, is an important issue in the legal world. The term, "conflict of interest," seems straightforward enough; however, the application of the concept is fraught with nuances that must be considered. While it should be obvious that you cannot work for the plaintiff and the defense at the same time, it isn't as clear that you sometimes may not work for more than one defendant in the same case.

Conflict of interest is an ethical issue for attorneys and, as such, is covered thoroughly in the American Bar Association's Model

Conflict of interest is an ethical issue...

Rules of Professional Conduct in Rules 1.7, 1.8, and 1.9. The General Rule, found in Rule 1.7(a), *says "A lawyer shall not represent a client if the representation of that client will be directly adverse to another client...."* 1.7(b) adds that *"A lawyer shall not represent a client if the representation of that client may be materially limited by the lawyer's responsibilities to another client or to a third person, or by the lawyer's own interest."* Although this speaks to the attorney's ethical responsibilities, it also applies to anyone involved in the litigation issues. LNCs also have an ethical code that speaks to this (see Ethics in Section 15).

The cases that every LNC must refuse

The conflict of interest impact on LNCs is particularly critical if the LNC continues to work in the clinical area. One shall not ethically take a case that is <u>against</u> the facility in which you work.   In addition, an LNC might even feel ethically uncomfortable in defending a case against the facility. Although in that situation, the ethical line is a bit harder to distinguish.

The offer of a contingency fee to consultants/experts is also considered unethical by the ABA as well as the AALNC. Contingency refers to doing the work and waiting for pay as a share of the proceeds after the case is won. No pay is anticipated by the plaintiff attorney if the case is lost (usually other than expenses). Plaintiff attorneys work on contingency fee in civil cases, taking 30 to 40% of the monetary judgment. After all, they have the responsibility of representing their clients "with reasonable diligence." The work done by an LNC is legitimate "expense" of the case preparation.   An LNC should NEVER consider a contingency fee, since it suggests that the consultant/expert might have been influenced to provide biased work product to help win the case.

A few conflict issues

❑   An LNC who does both plaintiff and defense work must keep impeccable records and carefully screen new cases for conflicts of interest with their existing cases/clients.

❑   An LNC who is personal friends with a physician might have to consider carefully whether or not to do a lawsuit either for plaintiff or defense in which the doctor is the defendant. Can personal knowledge or friendship be put aside to provide an unbiased review and assessment of the issues?

❑   An LNC who feels personal animosity toward a physician or facility might not provide an unbiased review either.

The Bottom Line

☑ Carefully consider your choices of specialty areas –your niche.

☑ Make a decision regarding whether to become a nurse expert witness.

☑ Recognize the value of medical/nursing expertise as compared to paralegal work.

☑ Conflict of interest is a continuing concern in the legal world.

Table 3-1 - Examples of behind-the-scenes consulting

❑ Review cases to determine merit before a lawsuit is brought.

❑ Review cases that are already filed, for either plaintiff or defense, to provide useful chronologies of the records and informative reports on the medical issues.

❑ Provide reports on research that may include specific standards of care or appropriate peer-reviewed journal articles or authoritative text references to support the medical issues involved.

❑ Locate information on, or actually obtain, appropriate expert witnesses for the case.

❑ Review medical records or other medical information for issues that have an impact on a legal matter.

❑ Organize and analyze medical records and determine missing medical records.

❑ Prepare reports, chronologies, time lines, medical fact issue reports, summaries, overviews, etc. regarding medical records and issues.

❑ Identify standards of care that relate to the case at hand and help in identifying causation and damages in medical malpractice cases or in product liability issues.

❑ Collaborate in developing strategies for medically related issues.

❑ Aid in preparing demonstrative evidence and exhibits for depositions and trial.

(Continued)

- Review medical files and provide informed support in workman's compensation or personal injury issues.

- Provide support in medical depositions—including preparing questions for same.

- Assist in developing settlement packages in regard to medical issues.

- Investigate issues and prepare reports regarding potential fraud related to health care providers.

- Review medical bills to determine over-billing, mistaken billing, misrepresentation, etc.

- Investigate potential medical misconduct by health personnel, often for the licensing boards of medical professionals.

- Investigate fraud and abuse of Medicare and Medicaid and other government funded agencies.

- Assess potential problem areas in hospitals, clinics, surgi-centers, etc. and provide risk management support and education.

- Provide life care planning or assessment of life care plans or vocational plans.

- Nurses with the appropriate background may assume the role of expert witness in nursing malpractice cases.

<u>Notes</u>

It does not matter how slowly you go,
so long as you do not stop.
Confucious

SECTION 4 - IDENTIFYING AND FINDING YOUR TARGET MARKET

dentifying and targeting potential clients in an efficient manner is the topic of this section. The more specifically you target potential clients, the more efficient you can be in utilizing those scarce marketing dollars.

MARKET WITH A RIFLE, NOT A SHOTGUN

Once you have chosen a specialty—or niche—you must then market to specific firms or groups that do that kind of work. This is called "marketing with a rifle." You aim specifically at your target market rather than using a "shotgun" approach of "scattering" your marketing resources. Specifically identifying your target market can save you money in marketing costs as well as prevent you from wasting your time and effort.

You don't just send a brochure to every law firm in the phone book.

You don't just send a brochure to every law firm in the phone book. Instead, learn to target those firms and individuals who are most likely to need your services and prepare your materials specifically toward their needs. You may choose more than one niche, but be sure to prepare and focus your marketing accordingly. This means adjusting the content of your marketing materials to be very specific. And you should <u>always</u> send your communications to a specific person—NOT "to whom it may concern." Adapting your marketing materials to specific clients is covered in *Section 7: Creating Effective Marketing Materials.*

> **Betty's Comment:**
> Just like physicians, lawyers can either be general practitioners or specialists. Many law firms specialize in real estate, corporate law, patents, probate, etc. They are poor targets for your marketing efforts.

FINDING CLIENTS IN THE MARTINDALE-HUBBELL LAW DIRECTORY

THE MARTINDALE-HUBBELL LAW DIRECTORY is published yearly in multiple volumes that cover attorney listings for every state. M-H Directories are usually found in law libraries, and Martindale-Hubbell information also is found on the Internet at **www.martindalehubbell.com**. Information about firms is listed by state, city, firm, and attorneys in the firm. The book directory and the Internet site are both good sources of information.

You can read the listed information about a firm and tell whether they do the type of cases that involve medical issues.

You can read the listed information about a firm and tell whether or not they do the type of cases that involve medical issues.

Often you can tell whether they do plaintiff or defense work by looking at the "Statement of Practice" and the "Firm Profile" (the Firm Profile is not included in every listing). If there is a list of "Representative Clients" at the end of the firm listing, look at the clients. Determine if the client list includes hospitals, insurance companies (personal injury OR medical malpractice insurance companies), or other facilities or corporations (products liability). Note that in the case of finding such "representative clients" listed, that this would indicate a defense firm.

You can also glean information such as how many attorneys are in the firm, what the specialty practice area is of each attorney listed, where they went to school and when, as well as get telephone and address information for the firm.

Knowing each attorney's legal specialty helps you select a name to whom you will specifically address your marketing materials. Be aware that you should get the latest set of Martindale-Hubbell since law firms have a way of "changing partners" and firm names as well as attorneys moving from one firm to another. Even with the latest set, we suggest you call to verify that the attorney is still there.

> **John Sez:**
> Martindale-Hubbell is a better source then your telephone book's Yellow Pages. Finding potential clients in the Attorney listing section of the Yellow Pages is a lot like picking through the 75% off sale table at K-Mart. You may have to sift through a lot of junk to get to the keepers.

LOCAL BAR ASSOCIATION LISTS

There are several ways to determine whether your county/city has a bar association. The local bar association may be listed in your phone book, or you may contact your local Chamber of Commerce for the information. Once you locate information on local bar

Hot Tip:: Some LNCs contact the bar association about making a presentation at one of their meetings.

associations, contact the bar association office to obtain information about its members and meetings. The MARTINDALE-HUBBELL LAW DIRECTORY also has a volume that contains listings for State Bar Association Profiles. Your local Chamber of Commerce also may have a list of attorneys in the area. Of course, you also can find a list of attorneys in your Yellow Pages, but it doesn't give you much information about what they do in the way of specializing—and that puts you back to "shotgun" marketing.

John Sez:

Joining your local Bar Association is an excellent idea. When you attend their meetings, workshops, and other events you get an opportunity to schmooze with attorneys in their natural habitat (we're talking "fox in the hen house" here). You will get plenty of opportunity to give the 30 second introduction that you are going to learn about in Section 9 of this guide.

JOIN THE RIGHT ORGANIZATIONS

.Joining the AALNC—the American Association of Legal Nurse Consultants—puts you in contact with other nurses who are involved in this field. You can learn a lot from your peers in LNC work. Some may work full-time with plaintiff or defense law firms; some will have independent practices; some may work for hospital risk management; some may work for insurance companies.

.Joining the AALNC... puts you in contact with other nurses who are involved in this field.

You can get good information about what they do and how they got started. Often these peers will know of job openings or of needs for contract work. They can also tell you about some of the local law firms and attorneys. This source often can be as good as using the MARTINDALE-HUBBELL. And, certainly, the programs offered at the AALNC meetings can be quite informative as well as providing continuing education credit at times.

Betty's Comment:
AALNC local chapters can be found in many large cities. Check _www.aalnc.org_ for a chapter near you. A requirement for membership in a local chapter is that you are a member of the AALNC national organization.

You can also join TAANA—The American Association of Nurse Attorneys. They are attorneys, but, of course, they are also nurses. You may not get much work from this group, since many do the same work you do, but it never hurts to get to know them. Their programs also can be instructive for you.

You can join a section of the ABA—specifically the Tort section. This may be of interest to you in that you can be kept up-to-date on many legal issues. You may also be able to attend local bar associations and seminars with greater ease and credibility. There are numerous benefits of the Tort Section of the ABA—your membership includes several journals and other informative materials.

Joining your local Chamber of Commerce or other local community group can sometimes be of benefit in getting your name and services before the community leaders, some of whom will surely be attorneys. This may be very helpful for your local area. Keep in mind though, that you may wish—or need—to market beyond your own community.

KNOW YOUR MARKET

The point of targeting your market means that you know who and where your market is. Know not only who is out there but

Knowing your market also helps you in knowing what kinds of problems they may have that you can help to solve.... also what they specifically do. Know where they went to law school; how old they are; what they specialize in; whether they are a partner or an associate. The M-H Directory is one source of this information. The M-H Directory will indicate whether they are a partner or an associate—there are two alphabetical listings of attorneys under firm names. The first listing is of the partners of the firm and the second listing is usually headed by "Associates." You can then send your marketing information to the person who has a reason to be interested in what you do. Usually, it is preferable to send your information to the partners of the firm who appear to be potential users of your services. It is important to know that final decisions are usually up to the partners.

DON'T LIMIT YOUR GEOGRAPHY

Many LNCs make the mistake of thinking their market is only the town, or section of town, in which they live. This is not necessarily so. Some LNCs are quite successful in carrying on a home-office based practice that serves clients throughout their entire region or state. Many of them have never met some of their clients face-to-face. Others make occasional forays into

Many LNCs make the mistake of thinking their market is only the town, or section of town, in which they live. other geographic areas to meet with clients or prospective clients, speak at bar association meetings, or attend legal conferences. Because of this networking, they end up with clients that are located far away from the LNC's base of operations. As your client base grows, you will be getting referrals from your existing clients. You too may end up with clients you have never met face-to-face.

Between the modern telephone network, the Internet, e-mail, USPO, Fed Ex, and UPS, it is possible to conduct a consulting practice from a cabin in the woods as long as you have access to reliable telephone and delivery service. Think of it this way: The bigger the pond you fish in, the more chance that you will actually catch a fish.

> **John Sez:**
> Limiting your geography is one of the most serious mistakes I see LNCs making. Think of the many small town law firms that exist with not an LNC in sight. Cultivating law firms in out-of-the-way areas may be a strategy you should consider.

THE INTERNET AS A MARKETING RESOURCE

Using the Internet to search for prospective clients can be efficient and is growing more useful every day. There are MANY sites on the Internet that can be useful to an LNC. However, this guide only mentions a few of the ones that can be used for locating information about attorneys. As already mentioned, MARTINDALE HUBBELL DIRECTORY is online. You can go to their web site at www.martindalehubbell.com or go to the web site of the American Bar Association at www.abanet.org which uses the Martindale-Hubbell database for searching for attorneys' names.

The Association of Trial Lawyers of America, or ATLA, which is a plaintiff attorney association, has a searchable web site as well. Their web address is www.atlanet.org. They have a stringent Use Agreement for searching for attorneys on their web site. Don't try to get a

...the Martindale-Hubbell book is the best source for learning as much as you can about attorneys...

long list of names from it, since it might appear that you are planning to solicit from them—and that is forbidden in their Use Agreement. You can use the ATLA web site to locate plaintiff attorneys, but it doesn't give you information on what kind of plaintiff work they do. In my opinion (Nurse Betty), the Martindale-Hubbell book and web site are the best sources for learning as much as you can about attorneys and firms. Other web sites, which have information about law firms, are included in the references and resources in Appendix B

> **Betty's comment:**
> If you are already active on the web and visiting "legal info" web sites, chat rooms, and list servs, I would suggest that you mostly "listen." Trying to make a "hard sell" to attorneys on the web or to convince them of how smart you are by "chatting" may backfire. After all, you have not been able to review the records. In addition, you may provide "consulting" they need for which you never are paid.

Many people think they must have their own web site. While this is not a "no-no," a web page can be expensive and time-consuming to develop and keep current. If you do not plan to keep current and helpful material on you web site, there is little need to have one. You can be listed in other sources on the Internet without setting up a web site. Also, there are monthly fees that you would be required to pay to an internet service provider (ISP) to maintain your web site. At this time we *do not* recommend that LNCs use a web site as one of their primary marketing tools. Web sites are not currently a good use of your marketing dollars. Internet based marketing keeps growing by leaps and bounds, and our opinion on this is subject to change in the future.

> **John Sez:**
> You don't need a website but you do need web access and an E-mail address. This will cost about $20 a month. Don't even think of going into business without it.

Many lawyers are not that familiar with the web themselves. They would rarely expect to find you on the web; they can't even find you in the yellow pages! However, we are beginning to see law firms that have web sites. As part of your research about a firm, you may want to see if they have a web site and, if so, view it to see what you can learn. If a high percentage of the legal industry moves to web-based marketing, you may have to follow suit. However, at the present, this is not the case. Once you get your marketing going smoothly, you might consider sending an e-mail letter to a firm. However, we would recommend that you always follow up by sending your brochure and other information by snail-mail as well.

> **John Sez:**
> You may want to avoid contacting law firms that have pictures of ambulances, cervical collars, or $1000 bills as a major feature of their web page.

A CAVEAT

It is smart marketing to try to learn which firms already have a nurse on staff full-time. If you believe a firm might have an LNC already, it is appropriate to contact that LNC to let her know you are doing contract work. She may be your best source in that firm for getting overflow work. Some firms are so large they have several nurses who work with different "teams" of attorneys. Be considerate of your fellow LNCs and respect their position in a firm. You may find this out at your local AALNC meeting or by calling a specific firm and asking if they have a nurse or nurses on staff. Ask to speak to the nurse if you have an opportunity.

It isn't unheard of that a firm would have overflow work at a time when multiple cases are going to trial; however, an attorney is more likely to put your marketing material in the "round file" because there is already a nurse "in-house." The nurse consultant on staff may keep your marketing information with the future in mind. At the least, if you contact the LNC and make a friend of her, you may add an astute LNC to your network (see *Section 9–Networking as a marketing strategy*).

The Bottom Line

☑ Market with a rifle not a shotgun.

☑ Know where to find information about your target market and learn all you can.

☑ Consider joining a professional group.

☑ The geography of your market is bigger than you think.

☑ The Internet is a good source of information for marketing.

☑ A web site as a marketing tool is not currently an efficient use of your money.

☑ Access to the Internet for research has become a basic requirement for an LNC.

☑ Having an e-mail address is another basic requirement.

☑ Marketing to firms that already employ nurses may not be good use of your time or money.

Notes

Nothing in life is to be feared.
It is only to be understood.
Marie Curie

SECTION 5 – PROSPECTIVE CLIENTS (PROSPECTS)

This section contains a model that is designed to help you categorize potential clients. You will learn how to tailor your approach to each category. Using this model can put you miles ahead of your competitors.

WHERE'S THE ACTION?

Law firms, insurance companies, and risk management departments that already have LNCs as part of their staff are not the best targets for your mainstream marketing efforts.

Your goal is to find those attorneys who do not already have a nurse on staff.

While knowledge of and networking within these groups can be of help and interest to you, it is not usually a good source of contract work for your business. Your goal is to find those attorneys who do not already have a nurse on staff. You get this information by calling the law firm you have researched and asking the receptionist (or whoever answers the phone when you call) if they have a nurse on staff. If you find out that the firm uses a nurse, but does not have the nurse as part of their employed staff, it is still acceptable to market that firm. You must realize however, that you will have to do better work than the LNC they are already using to get their business. Since you are new to this business, this will be difficult at first.

Betty's Comments:
Attempting to get work by undercutting the fee charged by another LNC is not helpful to you or legal nurse consulting as a whole. This may come back to haunt you in the future. Every time the firm has a case, they might pit you against another LNC who will "do it cheaper." Your work quality and dependability should set you apart, not how cheaply you will do case. Make your work efficient as well as good and the client will get an excellent work product for a reasonable price because of your efficiency. However, efficiency most often comes from experience of doing cases and developing an understanding of how to grasp issues clearly and express them succinctly.

With insurance companies and risk management departments, you are sure to find some nurses involved. In these cases, you might still be able to arrange a bit of contract work; however, some previous experience in cases is preferable to set you apart from others who have the same idea. The action, then, is to be found more often in those attorneys and law firms that you have researched (including the determination of whether they have an LNC on staff) and determined that they do the kind of legal work that involves medical issues.

MOST LNCS ARE NOT EFFECTIVE MARKETERS

When you realize how very few LNCs are effective marketers, it becomes clear that a tremendous opportunity exists for you to cultivate new clients. And best of all, there is less concern about competition from other LNCs since most of them don't have a clue about how to even categorize prospective clients, let alone have a plan to go after them.

THE HIERARCHY OF PROSPECTS

There are three types of prospective clients for your consulting services. We have named them **Hot Prospects**, **Aware but Unconvinced Prospects**, and **Unaware Prospects** (see figure 1 on the next page).

Hot Prospects make up a very small percentage of the market for your services. This means that the largest percentage falls

Hot Prospects make up a very small percentage of the market for your services.

into either the Unconvinced or Unaware categories. How that 99% splits out is highly dependent on geography.

Arizona, California, Florida, Texas, Pennsylvania, New York, and the Washington D.C. area have higher numbers of

...Arizona, California, Florida, Texas, ... and the Washington D.C. area have higher numbers of attorneys and law firms that are aware that LNCs exist

attorneys and law firms that are aware that LNCs exist. There are more LNCs in these areas, and they have opened up the market for you. This is a good

thing, since they have already been instrumental in educating attorneys in general about what LNCs can do for them. Other areas of the country are beginning to become aware of LNCs as well. This recognition will continue to grow as more LNCs develop their expertise.

Another general rule is that the larger the city the more likely that the legal establishment is aware that LNCs exist. This coincides with the fact that there are many more attorneys in the larger cities.

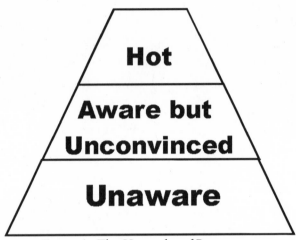

Figure 1 - The Hierarchy of Prospects

HOT PROSPECTS

Hot Prospects are attorneys, insurance companies, etc. that already recognize what an LNC can do for them, have a case or other work waiting, or may be

...Hot Prospects are trying to find you!

actively searching for an LNC to help them. These Hot Prospects are trying to find you!

The best thing that could happen to you in this case is to have impressed a Hot Prospect with some excellent work that you have done for them in the past. Alternatively, they may have seen an excellent presentation by you—including work samples —about your services. Consequently, you are the one who comes to mind when they start searching for someone to handle their case.

The next best thing that could happen is that you met this attorney sometime in the past and gave him, (1) your 30 second introduction, (2) your business card, (3) mailed him a card for his Rolodex®, and (4) a brochure which he filed for future reference. If you were sufficiently effective in making an impression, whom do you think he will call when a medical case arises?

Sometime, it seems that a Hot Prospect "falls" into your lap out of pure happenstance. Although that occasionally happens, it cannot be counted on as a significant marketing approach. More often than not, happenstance is like luck - you make your own. Likely, some word-of-mouth referral or learning about you from a reliable source has been the impetus for their calling you—and YOU had something to do with that.

...happenstance is like luck – you make your own

An attorney "Hot Prospect" that you have not met or sent marketing materials to may have heard about you from another attorney's recommendation. It still took your marketing skills and history of excellent work for another client to consider making that referral, even if it came in an indirect way.

> **John Sez:**
> Hot Prospects are trying to find you. They need your services. With a little luck and a lot of preparation, you will occasionally get a call from one of these. Hot prospects are as rare as a man who likes Tupperware parties.

AWARE BUT UNCONVINCED PROSPECTS

Prospects who are aware of LNCs, but are unconvinced, recognize that an LNC could possibly help them but haven't made the decision to actively seek one. Often this is because they have misconceptions about exactly what an LNC can do for them or how much it will cost. (Refer back to Section 3

> *Attorneys have misconceptions about exactly what an LNC can do for them or how much it will cost.*

about the difference between the behind-the-scenes consultant and the nurse expert witness.)

Sometimes these prospects know what LNCs do, but may not know how to go about finding one. It is even possible that they have met, or been contacted by, an LNC in the past but were under-whelmed by the experience.

Aware but Unconvinced Prospects represent an opportunity for you to make a positive impression that will move them to actively seek YOU when the need arises. This will take all of your marketing acumen since these prospects may not necessarily see a good reason to use the services of an LNC, and they often think they know~erroneously~what an LNC has to offer in a case.

When a prospect tells you they know what an LNC does, it is not a signal for you to back off. After all, they don't know what YOU have to offer. Obviously, it is important that you are aware and conversant about all the ways you can be of help to an attorney.

Your primary mission is to educate the prospect about the services you have to offer and how you can make a significant

> *Your primary mission is to educate the prospect about the services you have to offer [for]... solving their problems*

contribution to solving their problems. If some remedial education—vis-à-vis what an LNC really does—occurs as a result of your discussions, so much the better. Remember to approach them from the needs-based point of view. However, don't insult them by inferring they don't know or understand medical issues—use finesse in educating them and convincing them that you can be of benefit.

> **John Sez:**
> **Unconvinced is not the same as unconvincable.**

UNAWARE PROSPECTS

The chart indicates that "Unaware" prospects form the base of the hierarchy. This is where the greatest number of potential clients resides, and thus where you will have to spend a good part of your marketing time and dollars to educate these prospects. Unaware prospects could benefit from your services but do not have a clue that LNCs even exist. They require more convincing through multiple contacts with well-done educational (about LNCs) materials. However, once convinced, they can become good clients. They then become members of

Unaware prospects... do not have a clue that LNCs even exist.

that group of prospects who know you, know where to reach you, and know what you can do for them. In essence, you are moving them into the "Aware, but Unconvinced Group"—or even into the "Hot Prospect" group. Unaware prospects will need two types of training: (1) what an LNC does and; (2) what you can offer in the way of solutions to their problems.

Be clear about what types of services you offer and be specific about making linkages of those services to their problems. Remember the "show and tell" process of children. "Show" the attorney by letting them see the type of report you can provide as work product as well as presenting your brochure, and "tell" them, in an interview situation if possible, how you can specifically help them solve their problems. (See Section 11, Meeting with Prospects, for further discussion on this.)

The Bottom Line

☑ Understanding the hierarchy of prospects is critical to your marketing efforts.

☑ Most LNCs do not know about this model. This gives you a head start.

☑ Recognize that not all attorneys know about LNCs.

☑ Be able to "categorize" your marketing contacts after talking with them.

☑ Helping potential clients understand what you can do for them is the first hurdle you must overcome.

☑ One of the main purposes of your marketing materials will be to educate about LNCs.

☑ Tactful repetition of your marketing efforts is critical to your success.

Obstacles always show up when
you take your eyes off the goal.
Publilius Syrus (circa 43 B.C.)

SECTION 6 – HOW TO TURN PROSPECTS INTO CLIENTS

This section identifies those things that stand between you and your potential client. It discusses the expected results that your efforts should yield and provides a four-step process for turning prospects into clients.

MARKETING IS A NUMBERS GAME

Marketing your services is a numbers game that starts with targeting large numbers of prospects who have a high probability of having a case with medical issues. General marketing statistics tell us that only 1% to 2% of the potential clients targeted with direct mail respond. This means that out of 100 calls or mailings, you are doing well if one or two prospects respond. It is a waste of time to target attorneys and law firms that specialize in real estate, corporate, patent, bankruptcy, or tax law. Instead, go after attorneys and firms that practice in the areas of products liability, medical malpractice, personal injury, insurance defense, and workers compensation. This is why it is important to identify your market correctly—as noted in *Section 4- Identifying and Finding Your Target Market.*

A 1% to 2% response rate is the norm in the direct-mail business.

THE FOUR STEPS STANDING BETWEEN YOU AND YOUR CLIENTS

In order to get a client's business, four items must be present. A client must: (1) have a case with medical issues, (2) recognize that an LNC might be able to help, (3) think of you, (4) have a way to contact you.

The four items are, in reality, a four step process; failure at any one of these steps means that you lose the opportunity to consult. On the other hand, the more potential clients you market to, the greater the odds are that one of them will get through all four steps.

Think of the four steps as an endurance race with many runners (potential clients) starting at step one and finally a few making it to step four. It is obvious that the more runners starting the race, the better the odds are that some will reach the fourth step.

Step #1 – The prospective client must have a case with medical issues

Step #1 is obvious—there must be a case with medical issues. In fact, the issues must be significant. Many attorneys (and their paralegals) are quite comfortable handling the medical aspects of many types of cases. Be careful in this area; it is easy to insult a potential client by assuming they know nothing about the medical arena. A big part of your marketing job is to convince the client that you have specialized knowledge and skills that come with the experience of having worked in the medical environment - which, of course, is true.

Educating the attorney

Many attorneys think only in terms of using a nurse consultant for medical malpractice cases that involve nurses—and then only in terms of using the nurse as an expert witness. Nurses who think the same way compound this problem. LNCs work behind-the-scenes on all kinds of cases with medical issues, not just those that involve nurse practice issues.

Most medical malpractice lawsuits do not involve nurses. In the majority of med mal cases, the treating physician is the major focus of the case.

Attorneys may also think that you can help only in your specific area of nursing expertise such as OB or orthopedics. Nothing could be further from the truth.

Additionally, the issues in drug or medical device-related products liability cases (such as Fen-phen and breast implants) often benefit from having an LNC do medical literature research and reviews of records. Personal injury cases benefit by having the LNC review for potential pre-existing conditions or to help show or refute the causation aspects of the injury. There are even occasions for LNCs to be involved in criminal or family practice cases.

In educating a potential client, your first job may be to overcome this mind-set by helping them understand the full range of services that an LNC can provide. Having samples of your work product is a way of showing attorneys what you can do. Your marketing materials should also provide education.

Step #2 - They must recognize that an LNC is able to help them

Step #2 is all about educating the client. It is up to LNCs—individually and in groups—to educate potential clients about

Your potential clients must be educated on the various services that you provide...

the various types of legal cases in which LNCs can lend their expertise. Your potential clients must be educated on the various services that you provide as part of your practice. Telephone calls, face-to-face meetings (marketing visits), work samples, your brochure, cover letter, and other materials are all major educational and marketing tools.

Other ways to educate attorneys is to speak to attorney groups; write articles for local—or larger—legal papers or magazines; send an informative newsletter to your current clients as well as your prospects; do pro bono work. (*See Section 14–Other Low-cost Marketing Strategies* for further discussion of these methods).

Step #3 - They must think of you

So, you have cultivated a group of potential clients that do medically related cases, and you have spent some effort and

How are you going to get them to remember you...?

energy to teach them what you can do. As frequently happens, at the time you make your

contact they may not have a case for you to work on. How are you going to get them to remember you when the need arises? Again, this is a bit of a numbers game. Consider the following scenarios:

LNC #1: Mails a business card to a law firm.

LNC #2: Mails a business card and a brochure to a law firm.

LNC #3: Mails a business card and a brochure to a specific member of a law firm that she has researched in Martindale-Hubbell.

LNC #4: Mails a cover letter, a brochure, and a business card to a specific member of a law firm that she pre-screened using Martindale-Hubbell. In the cover letter the LNC mentions that she will be following up with a phone call in a few days to see if there are any questions about the information that was sent.

LNC #5: Mails a cover letter, a brochure, and a business card to a specific member of a law firm. The brochure includes a picture of the LNC. In the cover letter the LNC tells them she will be following up in a few days to see if they will grant her a 15 minute appointment. The purpose of the appointment is to come by and meet them and show them some samples of work product that will illustrate how you can help them with their medically related cases.

LNC #6: After doing #5 the LNC actually gets an appointment. She arrives professionally dressed and with a box of goodies for the office (doughnuts, granola bars, flowers, etc. see *Section 11– Meeting With Prospects* for a discussion on the power of goodies). She takes the time to meet the receptionist and the secretaries or paralegals (depending on the firm size, you may not be able to meet everyone). She meets with the potential client; listens to his problems; shows him some of her work samples that are relevant to the client's problems; goes over her brochure to help him understand the services she offers and how those services can give the client an edge over his opponents in a case. She leaves them with several copies of her brochure, business card, and Rolodex® card (one to keep, one to share). At the end of the interview, she asks the potential client "who else do you know that needs to hear about my services?" A day after the interview she sends them a follow-up thank you note for sharing their time with her. If the LNC doesn't hear from the client within 4-6 weeks, she sends an article that relates to an issue discussed during the interview.

...which of the six LNCs have the best chance of being remembered when the client has a need?

Considering the above scenarios, which of the six LNCs have the best chance of being remembered when the client has a need? Actually meeting with a potential client is a very big plus. It gives the client a chance to put a face with a name, and it gives you an opportunity to establish your credibility as a knowledgeable professional. People in all walks of life tend to prefer to do business with those they know and are comfortable with. The legal world is no different.

John Sez:
We are exaggerating in this section to make a point. The more of this stuff you do, the better your chances of having someone think of you when they need services of the type you provide.

Step #4 - They must have a way to contact you

Above we referred to brochures, business cards, Rolodex® cards, etc. All of these items are designed to (1) help the client understand what you do, (2) help them remember you, and (3) help them find you when they have a case for you.

Your objective should be to make it as easy and convenient as possible for a client to find and contact you.

Your objective should be to make it as easy and convenient as possible for a client to find and contact you. The quality of your materials speaks volumes about who you are and what you do. Quality materials are the first step in building the client's trust and confidence that your work product also will be of high quality. Quality includes actual "materials" (paper quality, design, etc.) as well as error-free and clearly stated content.

YOUR INTERFACE WITH THE WORLD

Some LNCs are quite successful in carrying on a home-based practice. Between the modern telephone network, the internet, e-mail, the post office, FedEx and UPS, you can conduct a consulting practice from any location. Several items concerning your interface with the world require your close attention.

Who answers your phone and how they answer it has a big effect on the professional image you want to present. Spouses, teenagers, and babysitters should be trained to take messages in a courteous and professional manner. They must be taught to get the correct information and a return call telephone number. However, having a separate line for business is <u>much</u> more professional and really gives the impression that you are in business and not playing around with a sideline.

Kids, dogs, and answering machines

Let's talk about your telephone image. Many full and part-time LNCs use their home phone number as their primary business number. This is not the best method—as suggested above— however, in the beginning, you may need to do this for cost-efficiency. Some issues to consider which may send a less than professional message are:

—cutsey answering machine greetings recorded by your kids;

—answering machine greetings that are designed to ward off tele-marketers and other assorted evil beings;

—any other kind of novel or less-than-professional sounding greeting.

> **John Sez:**
> Telecommuting lends itself to LNC work. A combination of a main telephone line for receiving client calls, a second line for making outgoing calls, faxing and accessing the internet is a basic essential in putting up the appearance that you are a serious business.

Your business telephone number

Many local phone companies offer the inexpensive option of adding a second telephone number to your existing telephone line. The second number rings with a distinctive ring. Thus, you know when the call is from a client rather then a personal call. The downside is that the phone company will not allow you to list that number as a business in the phone book. (However, that isn't really a downside, as noted below.)

As your business grows, you may consider getting a business line installed so that you can be found in the phone directory. The good news is that most phone companies will allow you to convert that second number to a business line number without forcing a number change on you. When you have a business number, all of the suggestions in the above section apply. You must answer the call in a business-like way and your answering machine message or answering service must be professional. You must remember to check your business messages regularly and return calls promptly. If you do not respond in a prompt manner, you may lose a potential client—and that client may be lost to all future work as well. The fastest way to turn off a client is to be slow or undependable in returning calls.

The fastest way to turn off a client is to be ... undependable in returning calls.

When you have a business line, you are listed automatically in the business Yellow Pages. This isn't all good. Often, there isn't an appropriate heading under which to place your listing. No one would think of looking for you under most of the headings that are in the Yellow Pages anyway. Even when you are in a small community telephone book, and they are willing to "add" a section, they are not usually willing to add one called "Legal Nurse Consultants." Besides, those attorneys who know little or nothing about LNCs are not likely to know where to look for that help and wouldn't know an LNC if bitten by one.

Nurse Betty, whose business is listed in the yellow pages, has had a number of "lay-people" call and want her to file something (legal) for them or to recommend a lawyer. Not a single attorney has ever called because of the Yellow Pages listing.

...a yellow pages ad is not recommended

For these reasons, we do not recommend a Yellow Pages ad. Even paying to have your name in bigger letters or in red is not worth the money, since your prospects won't be looking for you there, and your clients already know how to contact you.

> **Betty's comment:**
> My business has been listed under "legal support services" for about 5 years. I have had calls from the public and some from bonafide crack-pots—none of whom were lawyers.

The Bottom Line

☑ If only 1% to 2% of your marketing contacts respond to your efforts, you are having a great month.

☑ Prospects must have a case with significant medical issues before they actually need your help.

☑ The prospect must recognize that an LNC can provide solutions to their medical-legal case problems.

☑ The prospect must think of YOU and know how to contact you.

☑ Your telephone "persona" must always be professional, polite, and prompt.

☑ Two telephone lines are the basic minimum.

The more you say, the less people remember.
Francois Fénelon

SECTION 7 – CREATING EFFECTIVE MARKETING MATERIALS

arketing materials stand in for you whether you mail them or personally hand them out. They are evidence of your attention to detail and ability to communicate. It is important to develop your materials with this in mind. This section specifically identifies, and offers guidance in developing, the basic items you need to market your services.

FIVE THINGS YOU NEED TO KEEP IN MIND WHEN CREATING EFFECTIVE MARKETING MATERIALS

Betty's comment:
The adage that "you never get a second chance to make a good first impression" starts with your marketing materials.

Quality counts

One of the primary goals of your marketing methods is to establish your credibility in the eyes of your clients. The look

The look and feel of your marketing tools are important

and feel of your marketing tools are important—the quality of the paper stock

you use, the font types, and layout design can go a long way in establishing your credibility. Many office supply stores will print very inexpensive business cards. Don't succumb to the temptation to get the cheapest materials in this area; your image is on the line.

Client-centered material is the key

All your marketing material should be client centered, with the focus on the prospect's problems and the benefits your services can provide. You, your background, or your company should not be the major focus of the material except in the ways that show how you meet a client's needs. Attorneys will not necessarily be impressed with a long list of the CEU courses you have taken in the last ten years. Mentioning your kids, dog, age, or hobbies does nothing to improve your business image.

Attorneys will not necessarily be impressed with a long list of the CEU courses...

Customizing your material increases it effectiveness

The effectiveness of your marketing increases significantly if you develop marketing materials geared specifically to a particular type of client. For instance, if you were a plaintiff personal injury attorney, which would be more persuasive, a brochure with general information about what an LNC can do for attorneys in general, or a brochure telling specifically what an LNC can do for a personal injury attorney who concentrates on plaintiff cases?

...develop marketing materials geared specifically to a particular type of client

Don't assume your material has to be brief

Don't assume that your material has to be brief to be read. Interested prospects will want to know the details of the services you offer to help solve their problems. Research has shown that multi-page marketing materials do better than single page ones.

Interested prospects will want to know the details of the services you offer.

You create desire by helping your prospect imagine actually getting the benefits you offer.

Betty's Comments:
On the other hand, lawyers are paid by the hour, and they don't want to spend a long time reading materials sent by everyone who solicits them. Make your cover letter succinct and your brochure a problem-solving gold mine that they want to keep.

For example: As you read the newspaper each day you scan over hundreds of advertisements by stores and companies offering their goods and services, most of which you have no need or desire to buy.

Unless you need a new refrigerator, you are not very interested in reading ads for refrigerators, no matter how many exciting benefits, no matter how low the price. However, if your old refrigerator has just died, you are very interested in all ads for refrigerators. In fact, you will probably read every word of the ad describing the features, cost, and price.

This is not unlike many of your prospects. On the day your letter arrives, an LNC may be the furthermost thing from the prospect's mind.

On the day your letter arrives, an LNC may be the furthest thing from the prospect's mind.

Your prospect has nothing on the front burner that would require an LNC and is not interested in spending a lot of time reading about one.

Therefore, the best action you can hope for in most casesis that they will put your rotary card in their Rolodex® file and file your letter, brochure, and card in a place where they can find it when the need arises. Actually, you should probably suggest all of the above in your letter. The P.S. section is a good place to do this since studies have shown that

.... studies have shown that people read the opening line of a letter first and the P.S. second

people read the opening line of a letter first and the P.S. second.

Desktop publishing is the key to inexpensive customization

If you own a computer (PC or Mac), a <u>laser printer</u>, and have either Microsoft Word, Microsoft Office, Microsoft Publisher, Corel WordPerfect, CorelDraw, Microsoft Works, Adobe Pagemaker, or similar software, you can create first class marketing materials for a fraction of what professionally printed brochures and business letterheads cost. This is called "desktop publishing."

John Sez:
If you only have one printer it should be a laser printer. Ink jet printers are nice for color but the quality for documents and letters is noticeably inferior, and less professional looking, compared to output from a laser printer.

It is very easy to develop marketing materials that target specific clients by using desktop publishing. Desktop publishing programs allow you to develop a basic template for your materials and then modify them specifically to target potential clients on a one-prospect-at-a-time basis. This eliminates the cost of having hundreds of a standard, all-purpose brochure printed at one time leaving you no opportunity to tailor your materials to various markets. It is also helpful if your phone number or area code, etc. change, and you must change your materials.

There is nothing wrong with seeking professional help in designing your basic marketing materials. It is, however, expensive to use professional help. We have provided an example and general guidance in this section as well as in appendix B. Our point in this book is to help you develop "low-cost" marketing materials. However, if you do not feel comfortable in developing your own brochure in desk-top publishing, by all means, get professional help.

Some print shops offer design help. There are professional

...you need to be in control of the content of your materials

brochure designers offering their services as well. Our only caveat is that you need to be in control of the content of your materials. Not that you shouldn't follow the advice of the professional, but who understands what you do better than you?

THE TOOLS INDEPENDENT LNCS NEED TO MARKET THEIR SERVICES

There are several types of printed material that LNCs can use to promote their services. These include rotary (Rolodex®) cards, business cards, brochures, letters, work product samples, and newsletters. This section addresses all of these. (Appendix B contains examples of brochures and cover letters, feel free to steal all the ideas you like.)

Rotary Cards (Rolodex®)

There are several choices for rotary cards. The quickest and easiest is a **Business Card Insert Strip** made by Rolodex® that allows you to create an instant rotary card by inserting your business card into the strip. These cost around $5 for 40 of them and are available at most major office supply chains.

Avery's **Laser Rotary Card** (Avery #5385) can be used for desktop publishing your own rotary cards. These are an inexpensive approach to having a rotary card but must be done with care, since they can look unprofessional. A box costs $17.99 and will yield 40 cards.

Paper Direct offers a rotary card option on some of their more popular styles of brochures. The rotary card is perforated and is a part of the brochure. The brochure recipient has the option of removing the rotary card from the brochure.

While the Avery rotary card and the Paper Direct rotary card/brochure are options, neither produces the quality we would prefer. Consider having rotary cards printed or use the clear plastic business card insert strip by Rolodex®.

Business Cards

Your business cards should reflect a high level of quality and good taste. The advantage of desktop publishing business cards is that if addresses, phone numbers, or fax numbers change you can immediately update your business cards. The disadvantage is that most of the card stock used in desktop publishing is usually of insufficient quality. We recommend that you have your business cards printed professionally and ensure that you choose a good quality card stock. Your business card is such an important part of your image we do not think it is a place to "save a few bucks" by economizing.

We recommend that you have your business cards printed professionally…

Has anyone ever given you a card on which they had to hand-write changes? Were you impressed? Get them reprinted!!

Ten tips that will make your business card a standout

1. A short bulleted list of the main services you offer makes your card a mini-brochure.

2. E-mail addresses are appropriate provided that you check your e-mail regularly.

3. Your name should be in a larger type size then your address.

4. Your phone number should be located in the lower right-hand corner and of sufficiently large type to be read easily.

5. Adding a fax number increases your image as a serious business.

6. Be open to creative, but tasteful, alternatives such as a double sized card folded in half.

7. If using a double-sized folded card, adding a small, tasteful, head shot picture of yourself significantly increases the power of your card; however, attorneys rarely do this.

8. As you meet attorneys don't forget to ask for their card. Be sure and notice the style and quality of the cards you receive. You should strive for the same levels of quality and taste.

9. Restrain yourself from overdoing "fancy" fonts. Use simple, readable serif type for most of the card.

10. Use color carefully—both card stock color and font color. Simple is often more professional looking.

> **John Sez:**
> Just because you have Office Depot, Staples, Office Max, Kinkos or the like print
> your cards, it is not pre-ordained that you will be getting a "quality" card. They
> offer a wide range of card stock qualities. Look through their samples. Touch
> them, feel them, sniff them, gaze at them. It's your image, be picky about it.

Brochures

A well-designed brochure can teach, inform, and persuade.

The brochure is one of the LNC's primary marketing tools. A well-designed brochure can teach, inform, and persuade. It teaches a client how an LNC (you) can help them solve their problems. It informs them of who you are and extols the benefits, for them, of what you do. It persuades them to either call you now or keep your brochure in order to call you in the future when the need for your service arises.

A good brochure elicits action

The most effective brochures are designed to elicit one or more of the following actions:

❑   Call you to request more information

❑   Have a client call you with a case

❑   Call you for an appointment

❑   Be receptive for some future contact

❑   File the brochure so you can be contacted when the need arises for your service

The three most powerful things your brochure can contain

If you want to significantly increase the power of your brochure make sure it contains the following three items:

(1) Tell clients how you will solve their problems. One of the main reasons a client chooses to take action is that he or she has a problem that you are offering to solve.

LNCs who can recognize and solve problems succeed. Following are a few examples of brochure language that supports this approach. **(TIP: many of these make good bullet points in a brochure)**

> **Example 1** "Are you overwhelmed with medical records? Does your case have merit? Are your medical records complete? Do you need an expert? Are there pre-existing conditions that can become a bombshell in your case? Is there medical research available that will help or hurt your case?
>
> PSA Medical-Legal Services can help you answer these and other questions. We provide cost-effective case review, case analysis, and medical literature research in the areas of medical malpractice, products liability, personal injury, and Worker's Compensation. We provide the medical expertise you need to develop your strongest possible case."
>
> **Example 2** "PSA Medical-Legal Services provides the help and advice you need to...(good use of bullet points here) screen your medically-related cases for strengths and weaknesses; identify appropriate medical experts that can support your

case; summarize medical information in a form that helps you understand the issues; research the medical literature to ensure the appropriate research on the issues in your case."

Example 3 " PSA Medical-Legal Services can help you determine: The strength of a potential case; the issues that the opposition will most likely rely on; the standards of care that are most likely to apply in your case.

We offer analysis of the medical issues to help you determine the most appropriate strategy. We also can provide the necessary medical literature research to support the issues in your case."

(2) **Focus on benefits, not features, of your service**. This is sometimes a surprise to nurses who are new to marketing. The tendency is to elaborate on the features that make you look good, such as your background, your résumé, your curriculum vita (CV), your CEU list, or your methodology. Successful LNCs consistently use the 80-20 rule of communication. 80% of the brochure content focuses on the specific benefits you provide to your clients, only 20% is about you.

Successful LNCs consistently use the 80-20 rule...

Example 1 "PSA Medical-Legal Services offers the busy attorney a quick, cost effective method for understanding medical records. Protect your time and money by using our services."

Example 2 " PSA Medical-Legal Services can help you quickly determine what is, and is not, important to the medical issues in your case.

This saves you time, money, and, most importantly, keeps you from being blindsided by the opposition."

Example 3 " PSA-Medical Legal Services can help you quickly and thoroughly grasp the medical issues at stake in your case."

(3) Show that others value your services. Clients are willing to do business with you because they trust you. Listing other clients is a form of endorsement that increases the trust factor. This usually takes the form of a client list or some direct quotes from your existing clients.

Because a large part of your target market has little or no knowledge about LNCs, you MUST allot some of your brochure space to teaching clients about LNCs. As in the previous examples, this information is most effective when presented as solutions and benefits. (Note: A sample brochure is located in Appendix B.)

"...you MUST allot some of your brochure space to teaching clients about LNCs"

The process of developing your brochure

We have already mentioned the importance of quality paper stock in developing your materials. There are other important items to remember in the actual process of developing your brochure.

Be thoughtful in your choice of font or typeface. A serif font is preferred over a non-serif font. Serif refers to the little lines that occur at the top, sides, or bottom of the letter character—these make the font easier to read. A non-serif, or properly called, sans serif, font, usually is used only for headlines. Your word processing program should offer numerous choices of fonts.

Times Roman and Bookman are good fonts for the body of the text. Helvetica and Arial are two sans serif fonts often used. Stick with the more commonly used fonts for body text and headlines. Don't use flowing, script-like fonts—they are difficult to read. In considering the typeface, keep in mind also that ALL CAPS ARE HARD TO READ IN LARGE DOSES. Use all capitals only for headlines—and then only for IMPORTANT headlines.

Consider the size of the brochure and the way it is folded. There are several ways to fold even a tri-fold—for example, you can fold it in an accordion method or fold it over on itself. It is important to keep this in mind when you are determining the best place to put your name and contact information. You want that information to be easily found and easy to read. Plan your brochure so that the most important information is seen easily as the brochure is unfolded—or even when folded.

> **John sez:**
> We don't recommend doing a brochure to be mailed on its own. Our belief is that it should always be sent with a cover letter. Brochures mailed without an envelope are more likely to be tossed than are those with an attention-grabbing cover letter.

We can't state often enough—don't get "cutesy." If your style is always humorous, you may be able to develop a great brochure using humor. Paula Woo, a successful LNC in California and author of a humorous book on LNCs, has done this as well as any we have ever seen. She uses a humorous statement and a cartoon-type picture to get the attention. This fits Paula well, since her nature is to see the humor in life. However, her brochure is not hokum—it is professionally presented using humor. If your style is not naturally humorous, don't try to fake it in a brochure.

A well-designed brochure takes time and planning. It is your front line presentation is most cases. Consider brochure style, color, font typefaces, content, professional picture, and location of pertinent information carefully. This is an important part of you marketing materials.

Ten things you can do to enhance your brochures

1. Use good quality paper stock –at least 38 lb weight if possible.

2. Be sure your business and its contact information are clearly identified.

3. Humor only works when done extremely well—stick with the professional approach.

4. DON'T USE ALL CAPS – they are more difficult to read.

5. Use only one or two typefaces in a brochure, e.g., Arial and Times Roman. Use Arial for headlines and headings; use Times Roman for body text.

6. Bullet points are good; as are active verbs.

7. Your brochure is a good place to have your picture.

8. Don't use jargon—either medical or legal.

9. Follow the 80/20 rule.

10. White space is good; try not to clutter.

Cover Letters

It is always appropriate to send a cover letter with a brochure, card, or résumé. A letter addressed to a specific person is more likely to be opened and read. A cover letter is usually a short, one-pager and serves to "whet the appetite" of the reader to look at your brochure, save it, and possibly even give you a call. However, you are usually the one who must take the active role of further contact.

If you have met the lawyer through networking or had someone give you her name to contact, this is the first thing you refer to in your letter. If you have not met or been referred by someone, then your letter will need a different opening.

Beyond the use of a specific name, there are other important items to remember when writing your cover letter. The following pages suggest some specifics for writing good cover letters. (Appendix B also contains several examples.)

What it takes to get your letter read

Direct mail experts say that you only have 5 seconds to capture your prospect's attention. Only the first two or three sentences will be read to capture the purpose or interest of the letter. If you don't capture the interest in those lines, the letter will likely be tossed along with the brochure.

...experts say that you only have 5 seconds to capture your prospect's attention.

Don't be shy; use a strong opening line or even a headline to grab the reader's attention.

To hold your reader's interest, the body of your cover letter should contain the following:

❑ Start with an attention-grabbing opening sentence.

❑ Be succinct in stating your personal information—your brochure should cover that well enough.

❑ Only state enough to identify yourself for the purpose of the contact.

❑ Know about the prospect/firm to whom the letter is sent:
   —what their practice emphasizes (plaintiff or defense? Med mal? Personal injury? Etc.)
   —what their needs are (or might be, considering their practice)
   —how you can help meet those needs

❑ Close with a specific action identified
   —"I will call you..."

❑ Thank them for their consideration of your letter and brochure.

Examples of attention-grabbing opening lines:

Example 1: It was a pleasure to meet you at the Bar Association breakfast last Tuesday. As I promised, I am sending you the information about my services that can help you get a better control over and understanding of the medical issues in your cases. (For someone you have already met and spoken with—obviously)

Example 2: Winning cases with medical issues is more likely when you have the medical information at your fingertips in a well-organized, analyzed, and summarized format. As a nurse with many years of clinical experience, I can provide you the advantage of having your case medical records and information not only well-organized but also well-researched and interpreted. (This one and the next are possible openings when you are sending marketing materials out in a "cold call" fashion.)

Example 3: If you have ever had to deal with the confusion of disorganized medical records, you know how frustrating it is to find the meaningful facts you need for the case. As a nurse with many years of clinical experience, I can help you get the records organized and summarized for your efficient and informed use in litigation.

Notice that the above opening sentences address the prospect's needs and speak to what the LNC can do to solve the problem.

The second paragraph might say something about the firm— indicating you know what they do that you could be of help with. You might start the paragraph with something like:

"Since your firm does plaintiff medical malpractice, you are surely faced with the problem of determining which cases are viable for litigation purposes. I can review those myriad cases and cull out those with little or no merit and offer recommendations and research regarding standard of care on others that seem to have potential for litigation."

For a defense firm, you might say:

In your defense cases of (medical malpractice) (personal injury) (products liability), it is always difficult to know whether you have all the records and have them in an appropriately organized and summarized fashion. Or you may need to determine what type of expert would best serve the case and how to find the expert; I can help in both of those areas."

In your closing paragraph, we recommend that YOU take the active role by saying how you plan to follow up this letter. You might state that you will call them to make an appointment so that you can discuss how you might provide solutions to their problems related to medical issues. Experts recommend that you make the follow-up call no later than two or three days of the prospect receiving the letter.

Closing the letter by saying that you hope they will "call you if they have a case" or "call you if they want to know about your services" is a poor substitute for your taking action as a follow-up to your mailing.

John Sez:
The fastest way to destroy your image and credibility is to tell prospects that you will be calling them and then not follow up when it is time to call. I'm the first to admit that marketing yourself takes a certain amount of guts. However, no guts, no glory.
If you have what it takes to be a successful LNC, you must pick up that phone and call.

A caveat from Nurse Betty

In my experience in helping nurses prepare letters, etc. for their business, I have found a tendency of many nurses to want to say they are "cheaper than doctors." RESIST THE URGE! Don't even mention doctors in your letter or materials (except that one of the services you offer is finding physician-experts).

Most doctors do not even do the same thing for attorneys that

Most doctors do not even do the same thing for attorneys that you do.

you do. Doctors more often do a quick overview of a case and state an opinion about the issue(s). There is plenty of room for both an LNC and a doctor on a case.

The LNC (behind-the-scenes, of course) makes sure all the records are accounted for; organizes, and often paginates them, for ease of use by the attorney; summarizes them in some format (there are choices such as narrative or chronological or time line); and provides any needed literature research and explanation of the medical records.

Nurses can also help locate and interview potential physician experts as well as specialty area nurse experts. (Remember, nurses are only experts in cases with nursing issues.) Very few physicians offer these kinds of services, so avoid making comparisons.

In fact, if the attorney says he has a doctor who reviews his cases, ask if the doctor provides summarization and organization of the records or literature research.

The statement that you are "cheaper" than a doctor only holds true in the hourly rate (usually). The total project might show that your work product ends up costing more than the physician's short review.

There is a second part of this to consider, however. If the

...you CAN offer a less expensive solution for the attorney...

attorney does plaintiff medical malpractice and needs someone to determine merit in cases, you CAN offer a less expensive solution for the attorney—particularly in the "first pass" over the cases that come into a firm. You could do the initial review and decide which have potential and would benefit by having a physician review them.

It is also true that you often can provide literature research to support merit of any type med mal case yourself. This is another reason it is important for you to understand your role in LNC work as you get started in marketing your services.

Newsletters

Developing a newsletter to send to clients and prospective clients is a good marketing device. It is time-consuming, however, and requires careful consideration of content. To be more than

...filling up a page or two or four with medical jargon will not do...

just another piece of junk paper crossing the attorney's desk, you need content that speaks to the attorney's needs (where have you heard that before?). Just filling up a page or two or four with medical jargon will not do that; you need to consider the potential interest in and importance of the information to an attorney.

For example, if the attorney does personal injury cases, articles about back injury, whiplash, etc. will be of interest. A few years ago, an article in a well-known medical journal reported that a number of persons showed evidence of herniated discs on MRI though they had no history of trauma and no report of symptoms. The data from this were interpreted by some to indicate that some people, who claimed herniated discs after a minor incident, may fall into the category of having had the herniated disc prior to the injury—not caused by the injury.

The article itself proved nothing, but a personal injury defense attorney might find this information of interest and might find occasion to apply that theory in a given situation. Plaintiff attorneys, as well as defense, would find articles about fibromyalgia of interest since it is among the common complaints of personal injury clients and since there is still some controversy about this condition.

...attorneys...find articles about fibromyalgia of interest since it is among the common complaints of personal injury clients.....

Medical malpractice attorneys, either plaintiff or defense, might find updated information on breast cancer studies of interest. You might use a medical malpractice case reported in a local or national legal paper and then review some of the medical literature research on that issue. Obstetric cases are quite common and any new or updated information (even a good explanation of "old" information) that sheds any light on this type of case is usually well received.

Of course, one of the reasons for sending a newsletter would be to promote your services in these situations. However, this needs to be done in a way that isn't "in your face." A newsletter that is only—or mostly—about the LNC is recognized for what it is immediately—just a sales sheet. Make the newsletter worth reading and make the information about your services low key but specific.

...promoting your services... needs to be done in a way that isn't "in your face."

Newsletters used for marketing should be sent out more than once – different editions that is. In other words, try to put out a newsletter with some regularity—every quarter or every other month—not just as a one-time thing.

...try to put out a newsletter with some regularity...

As for the actual process of producing a newsletter, you can use the template in your word processing program or use a specific desktop publishing program like Microsoft Publisher or PageMaker. Paper Direct offers both preformatted newsletter paper and templates. Or, you might have someone do the newsletter for you; however, you should be the one who decides on the content and who makes certain the material is appropriate and correct—in content as well as presentation. As with your other marketing materials development, you should retain control of and input into any newsletter that is to be sent as part of your marketing.

Work Product Samples

It is highly recommended that you develop samples of your work product. If you have done any cases, **take the information and change it around so it will not be recognized;** use the ideas only for showing how you did a summary or a time line or a chronology, etc.

> **Betty's comment:**
> Many experienced LNCs advise that you should be very careful about using actual cases even though they may be "disguised." The only cases they are even close to comfortable with using in a sample are those that have already settled and are closed. Even then, the information about the plaintiff's medical record is still confidential. You should also disguise any hospital and doctor(s) involved as well as the patient.

Have these sample materials in your presentation folder when you interview with a potential client. A complete case chronology or report is not required—or even recommended. Show sample pages of various types of work product such as time lines, narrative reports, chronologies, etc. using different cases. It is NOT recommended that you give the potential client a copy of these samples—only show them the format and point out that you can provide that kind of work product support in their cases related to medical issues.

If you have not done any cases yourself, check with LNCs in your network to see if they will help you develop a work product sample. This requires a fair amount of work but is worth it if you can show the attorney rather than just telling (remember show-and-tell in school?). If you have taken an LNC course, you should have materials from which to develop your work product sample. You can also "make up" case information to use in a work product sample. You are not required to give case outcomes or total work products. These samples are only to show your ability to prepare information in different formats as preferred by different clients.   You might also consider showing a report on the medical research for an issue—and include at least an abstract in the sample.

It is understood that there should be no spelling errors, no typos, nor any other pitiful excuse of a less than stellar sample work product. The sample should be clean, correct, and professional. It should be on white paper and not have any frou-frou, either in the formatting or the paper. This is a work product, not a way to show what amazing things you can do with a computer or what darling paper you have found. This work product, even if it is only a sample, it is a representation of YOU AND YOUR PROFESSIONALISM.

> **John Sez:**
> Don't give away the store. We strongly advise against leaving work product samples with potential clients. The form and format that LNCs use to summarize medical cases may make a tempting model for an attorney to hand to a legal secretary or paralegal and say "use this as an example of how to do our cases." On the other hand, I will admit that after you do your first case for them, they will have the model. After doing a case for them, they should have a strong sense of the fact that you are adding value via medical expertise.

"TO RÉSUMÉ OR NOT TO RÉSUMÉ" THAT IS THE QUESTION.

We <u>do not</u> recommend that you include a copy of your résumé as part of your marketing

We <u>do not</u> recommend that you include a copy of your résumé...

materials. It can be a distraction from your real purpose, which is, to help the client understand what you can do for them and their problems—and your brochure is designed to do that. Attorneys seldom use their résumé as a marketing tool. Why should you be any different?

If the potential client wants your résumé, he will ask for it. This

If the potential client wants your résumé he will ask for it...

means that you must have a well-done résumé and keep it updated (constantly). Like all your other marketing materials, prepare your résumé in a professional manner. You do not need to have another "professional" do your résumé though. There are plenty of self-help books available with excellent examples of a good résumé.

An exception to the no-résumé rule:

The only strong exception to the no-résumé rule is for LNCs who want to do expert witness work. In that case, your résumé will be a well-developed curriculum vita (CV)—confirmation of the knowledge, skills, and experience that make you an "expert." A CV is usually a more extensive document than a résumé and includes details on any publications, talks, or other activities relevant to your expertise as a nurse expert witness. Whereas a résumé is usually no more than two pages, a CV may go on for many pages, listing all the relevant information of experience, publications, presentations, etc.

Nurse expert witnesses should spend the money and time to work with a professional résumé and CV writer to develop credible materials since so much of their business will depend on the professional image presented.

John Sez:
A Word to the Wise About Pictures Pictures can be a powerful addition to your marketing material. The picture helps put a name with a face and is another way of getting yourself in front of the prospect. A picture can be another way of helping prospects visualize who you are.
Do not succumb to the temptation to use "Glamour Shots," your prom picture, high school graduation picture, or a Polaroid shot by Uncle Harry. A professionally done picture is required for marketing. How can the client take you seriously if you don't take yourself seriously enough to offer a professional representation of yourself? Don't cheap-out on this one.

We like Paper Direct products

Paper Direct (800-272-7377), a printing supply house, offers a wide variety of color-coordinated brochures, business stationary, business cards, rotary cards, and newsletter formats that you can print on your laser printer. They also offer software templates for the most popular desktop publishing computer programs, such as PageMaker and MS Publisher, which enable you to create excellent professional brochures using Paper Direct's pre-printed paper stock. Their paper templates let you avoid spending hours measuring and laying out text. Paper templates have all the margins, borders, tabs, and boxes already set for each Paper Direct brochure, business card, etc. All you do is plug in your information.

It is possible to coordinate letterheads, brochures, business cards, envelopes, newsletters, and postcards in various styles. The best part about Paper Direct products is that they have been designed by professionals so that both the layout and the colors are optimized to make your materials look good. One caveat in using this or similar pre-colored designs is to carefully consider the impact you want to make. Although the designs are professionally done, some are not appropriate for your consulting business. Don't get flowery or frou-frou type papers—stick with professional looking materials. Additionally, the paper's "weight" may be too thin to connote quality. For a brochure, 38lb weight is more desirable then 28lb.

We have no association with Paper Direct except that we have used their products for many years and have been particularly pleased with both the quality of their products and their devotion to excellent customer service. There are similar paper products available at other companies, such as Beaver Prints (814-742-6070), and at office supply stores. Just be sure you get good quality paper, appropriate design, weight, and colors, and that you can get more of the same design as you need it in the future.

The Bottom Line

☑ You can significantly increase the chances of getting a client by focusing your marketing materials on the prospect's problems and the solutions you offer.

☑ Quality counts.

☑ Continue marketing with a rifle, not a shotgun, by customizing your material.

☑ Follow-up of marketing contacts is important.

☑ Desktop publishing is the key to low-cost, high impact materials.

☑ Use a laser printer for marketing materials, even if you must have someone else print it.

☑ Spend the time to develop a good cover letter.

☑ Work-product samples are an important part of your marketing package.

☑ Professionally done photographs are a welcome addition to your materials.

☑ Résumés are not recommended as part of your initial marketing package—but keep an updated résumé in case it is requested at any time.

☑ Nurse expert witnesses will need a well-done curriculum vita instead of a résumé.

Society is always taken by surprise
at any new example of common sense.
Ralph Waldo Emerson

SECTION 8 - WHAT YOU NEED TO KNOW ABOUT DIRECT MAIL

You can spend hours developing a great direct mail package, but your efforts are wasted if your prospects don't open the letter or if it is tossed in the trash by secretaries or administrative assistants before it reaches the prospect's desk. It is important to recognize that businesses receive a mountain of mail every day, much of it unwanted. The items in this section will increase the effectiveness of your mailings and, therefore, the chance that your mail will get read and by the right person.

WHY USE DIRECT MAIL?

Created skillfully, direct-mail advertising enables you to go through the entire selling process...

The purpose of direct mail in your LNC marketing is to pave the way for a visit to a prospective client's office. Direct mail allows you to take the most careful aim at your target audience. Created skillfully, direct-mail advertising enables you to go through the entire selling process—from securing your prospects' attention, to actually obtaining sales by means of telephone conversations and/or in-person meetings.

Brochures sent by direct mail offer the greatest opportunity to go into detail about your services. People expect a lot of information from a brochure, so feel free to give it to them.

Follow-up telephone calls, which you set the stage for in your cover letter, allow you to be even more specific. Used as an adjunct to direct mail, a follow-up call can generate a visit to a potential client's office.

Betty's Comment:
Remember that your marketing materials will be the first impression you make on this prospect and that "first impressions" carry a lot of weight. Always have correct, well-written, professional materials. I repeat myself about this issue purposely.

Successful LNCs are not fazed by the amount of direct mail

Successful LNCs are not fazed by the amount of direct mail assaulting their prospects every day.

assaulting their prospects every day. They know how to break through that barrier: with follow-up mailings, follow-up telephone calls, and follow-up visits. (Get the picture? Follow up, follow up, follow up.)

GETTING YOUR MAILING TO THE ACTUAL PROSPECT

Address your material to the right person

You should never send direct mail materials to a law firm using

You should never send direct mail materials to a law firm using only the firm's name as the primary addressee.

only the firm's name as the primary addressee. Doing this virtually guarantees that the mail will be opened by someone other than one of the firm's attorneys and most likely will be put into the round file (or oblong, as the trash can may be) immediately.

Use your Martindale-Hubbell information to specifically address an attorney by name and be very careful to spell the name correctly. It is helpful to cross-check your Martindale-Hubbell against your local phone book as an additional accuracy check. If doubt still exists, consider calling the law firm to verify the correct name, its spelling, and the proper address. Also remember that lawyers often change firms during the year, and it behooves you to be certain the lawyer is currently still with the firm.

Don't assume that sending it to a law firm gets all the members of the firm covered

Law firms are busy places, and the people working in them frequently communicate on an "as needed" basis. They each have their cases for which they are responsible and may work with other attorneys in other cases. However, they are unlike nurses who have "report" at the beginning of the day. Lawyers who are not working

lawyers ... do not take time to share information tidbits

on the same case do not take time to share information tidbits. Many firms are large and do their work in teams. One team is not likely to share information, such as your brochure, etc., with other teams.

Consequently, you should not assume, because you sent you marketing materials to a particular lawyer in a law firm, that anyone else in the firm has seen your information. Mail your material to each attorney in the firm that you think might have use for your services. This way it is more conceivable that at least one of them will see the benefit of the services you offer.

DEVELOP A DIRECT MAIL CAMPAIGN

To make direct mail work you need to use it with some regularity. You will have an informative brochure, business cards, rotary index cards, and a cover letter that you have planned and implemented with great care. Initially, you might want to send 10 to 20 sets of these marketing materials a week —no more than you can follow up with phone calls, and, with luck, visits within a few days after they have been received. Once you develop some ongoing clients, you will be able to spend more time doing legal nurse consulting and less on mailings and follow-up.

However, don't be fooled into thinking you can eventually stop your mailings altogether. This process is relatively ongoing if you want to keep enough business coming in. Remember, this is a numbers game. A 1% response rate is good. This means that you must keep a steady stream of mail in the pipeline. And you need to muster whatever courage it takes to make those follow-up calls.

... this is a numbers game. A 1% response rate is good.

Betty's Comments:
One of the greatest ways to undermine your integrity is not keeping your promises. Even though the recipient may only be a prospect, if you say in your letter that you are going to call but never follow through, what do you think the lawyer will do with your materials? If your answer was, "toss them," you are correct. And if that attorney ever needed a nurse to help in a case, you would not be the one called.

REPEAT THE MESSAGE

Have you ever noticed that Publishers Clearing House does not stop with one mailing? They send a steady stream of mail in hopes that sooner or later you will respond. You need to

...send a steady stream of mail....

follow the same concept. Although you don't need to be as obnoxious.

Don't be shy about sending your mailings to the same prospect more than once over a period of time. Repeating the message is a basic principle of advertising. And if you are sending repeat information, it certainly makes sense to have researched the firms and attorneys to whom you are sending it. Therefore, we reiterate a principle concept here, which is to "be informed about your clients and prospective clients."

Eventually, repetition has a subconscious effect. Most people are not aware that their opinions have been influenced, but it is

Eventually, repetition has a subconscious effect

common. Marketing studies have shown that even a person who thinks they are unaffected by an ad campaign still tends to pick out the familiar name when confronted with a choice between brands. Which brings us right back to a basic principle of LNC marketing, which is, "We are more comfortable with things we know and distrust the unfamiliar."

You should send follow-up packages at an interval of no longer than three to six months. After you have been at it a while, your weekly mailing should be 50% new names and 50% re-mailings to your researched list.

FISH IN A BIG POND

You must market in a big enough area to make the numbers game work. In the previous section, we alluded to the fact that it isn't necessary to conduct a face-to-face relationship with your clients. It is certainly appropriate and desirable to have at least an initial face-to-face meeting. However, most of the independent LNC's work can be, and usually is, done without the need for eye-to-eye interfacing. This is good news! It means that you can expand your client base well beyond your current geographic location. It is not unheard of for an LNC to have clients within a 100 to 200 mile radius. In some cases, clients are scattered throughout a state or across the country. This idea is critical to LNCs who live in small towns, rural areas, and cabins in the woods. All this requires is adapting a mindset that it can be done.

Seven Tips For Improving Your Mailings And Increasing The Chances That They Will Be Opened

1. For the business and legal environment, personalized business letters mailed in business sized letter envelopes work best. Do not be tempted to use bright colored or unusual envelopes.

2. Type the address on the envelope using either a typewriter or preferably, a laser printer. A poor second choice is to use a clear laser label. Do not address your envelopes with mailing labels unless there is absolutely no alternative.

3. Use standard, business style fonts such as Times Roman.

4. Mail first class using a stamp, not a postage meter. Stamped mail is more likely to get opened than metered mail.

5. Use high quality envelopes and letterhead stationery with your company name as the return address.

6. If you have a prime prospect and you want to absolutely, positively guarantee that your mail will be opened, send it by priority mail for $3.20, or via UPS, or Federal Express.

7. If you are mailing information in response to a telephone conversation or request for information, write on the outside of the envelope, "Enclosed is the information we discussed," or "Enclosed is the information you requested." This significantly improves the chances of getting past most gatekeepers and to the attorney.

The Bottom Line

☑ Marketing is a lot like fishing; the more bread you cast upon the water, the better the chances are that something will take the bait.

☑ Address your mail to a specific attorney, not the law firm in general.

☑ It is important to research the attorney/firm you are targeting.

☑ Mail your material to every attorney in a law firm that your research shows could use your services.

☑ You must develop an organized plan for your mailings and re-mailings.

☑ Fish in as big a pond as possible.

☑ REPEAT the message.

Notes

Practice what you know, and it will help
make clear what you do not know.
Rembrandt

SECTION 9 - YOUR 30 SECOND INTRODUCTION

This section introduces you to one of the most powerful marketing tools in your arsenal. Your 30-second introduction. The last thing you want to happen is for a potential client to ask you what you "do" and you respond with "I'm a nurse," or "I'm a nurse-consultant."

"HOW CAN I POSSIBLY EXPLAIN WHAT I DO IN THIRTY SECONDS?"

Your first response to a 30-second-first-meeting-introduction is likely, "You must be kidding!" However, once you think about it, a well-planned commercial *a well-planned commercial is no longer than thirty seconds* is no longer than thirty seconds, and is often shorter, but it gets the point across. If you can't "hook" someone's interest in thirty seconds, you may not have any further chance to "explain" what an LNC can do for a client.

This 30-second introduction not only is used with prospective clients but also with anyone who may have an interest in what you do. A 30-second introduction is just a "set-up" to give some pertinent information and lead the person with whom you are talking to ask further questions of you. It is a requirement when you are doing large group networking (see later section on networking).

How to develop the ideal 30-second introduction

Follow this four step process to develop the ideal introduction:

Step 1 – State who you are and who your company is (if you are operating under a company name) (*note that this only tells who you are—not what you do*)

Step 2 – Creatively tell what you do. (*If your introduction uncovers some interest, keep going to step 3 &4.*)

Step 3 – Ask one or more leading question

Step 4 – Follow-up with those who express an interest

APPLYING THE 4 STEP PROCESS

Step 1 - Who you are

Start your introduction with who you are. For instance:

"My name is Jane Smith, I'm a legal nurse consultant."

Or *"My name is Jane Smith, I'm a legal nurse consultant with PSA Medical Legal Services."*

Betty's comment:
Often, your name and the statement that you are a legal nurse consultant has already been part of the conversation. If that is the case, start with Step 2 and, at the appropriate time, tell what you <u>do</u>.

Step 2 - What you do

You must be able to state the gist of what you do in one or two clear sentences, so that anyone hearing can decide if they want to know more. Here is a handy matrix for developing step 2.

The "what-I-do" fill in the blanks matrix

Use this fill-in-the-blanks matrix as an aid in developing your "What I Do" statement. (Add or change the wording to suit your needs or the situation.)

I, or we, (Field 1)_____
 (Fill-ins: provide support for; help; work with; collaborate with)

(Field 2)_____
 (Fill-ins: attorneys; insurance companies; defense attorneys; plaintiff attorneys)

to (Field 3)_____
(Fill-ins: present the strongest possible medical case; develop a thorough understanding of the medical issues in their case; increase the chances of winning a medically related case; present medical issues in a well organized way; develop winning strategies in a medical case)

by (Field 4)_____ .
(Fill-ins: getting their medical information organized for them; clarifying medical issues so they can be understood and dealt with effectively; organizing the medical information and clarifying the issues for them.)

John Sez:
 Notice the 80/20 Rule is at work here, the greater emphasis is on attorneys' needs rather than who you are.

> ## Some examples of applying the "what I do" matrix
>
> ❑ "I work with attorneys to increase the chances of winning their cases by organizing the medical information and clarifying the issues for them."
>
> ❑ "I help attorneys to develop a thorough understanding of the medical issues in their case by clarifying the medical issues for them."
>
> ❑ "We support defense attorneys to develop winning strategies in a medical case by getting their medical information organized and clarified for them."
>
> ❑ "We collaborate with plaintiff attorneys to reduce case preparation costs by quickly and efficiently getting their medical case issues organized for them."

If your introduction uncovers some interest keep going to steps 3 & 4

After you have given your succinct, 30-second introduction, you should be able to tell if you have elicited any interest. If you don't note any interest, then you might just give them a card and move on. If there is some interest shown, then follow up with steps 3 and 4. Note that Steps 3 and 4 are actually intermingled—not necessarily one following the other.

Step 3 - Ask leading questions

After you creatively say what you do using your 30 second introduction, and your conversation partner has shown an interest, ask a leading question or series of questions that makes the prospect think and respond in a way that gives you needed information. (The questions must be open-ended in order to get the prospect thinking and talking, not merely answering yes or no. Recall your psychiatric nurse interview training.)

The leading questions are a critical step in your introduction, because they help you classify the prospect as a potential client and set up your response about how you can help them specifically.

The needed information you are looking for falls into two categories; (A) general questions that tell you that this is a potential client for your services, and (B) specific questions that tell you in what areas the client could potentially use your help.

There is no reason to tell a prospect how you can help until you have uncovered what kind of help (if any) he or she needs.

Formulating leading questions

When formulating your leading questions ask yourself this:

❑ What information do I want to get as a result of asking this question?

❑ Can I include or exclude this person as a prospect as a result of this question?

❑ Does it take more than one question to find out the information I need?

❑ Do my questions make them think?

❑ Can I ask a question that separates me from my competitors?

❑ Does this question help me categorize this person in the hierarchy of prospects?

❑ Have I phrased my question so that it doesn't seem abrasive or intrusive?

Some examples of (A) general leading questions

❑ *"What is your biggest problem with medical issues?"*

❑ *"What type of medically-related cases do you usually encounter?"*

❑ *"What experience have you had with legal nurse consultants?"*

Some examples of (B) specific leading questions

Limit yourself to <u>one or two</u> of the following questions:

❑ *"What type of medical expertise do you usually rely on?"*

❑ *"What do you find to be the most difficult part of preparing a medically related case for trial or settlement?"*

❑ *"What other attorneys or law firms do you know that use legal nurse consultants as their secret weapon?"*

❑ *"How do you currently organize and summarize a large pile of medical records?"*

❑ *"Who do you use to research the literature regarding medical issues?"*

❑ *"What do you do about reviewing cases for merit?" (if plaintiff attorney)*

Ask enough leading questions to gauge interest in your services

You should ask just enough questions (type A and/or B) to see if the person is listening and really interested in what you do.

...ask just enough questions (type A and/or B) to see if the person is listening...

Remember, at many gatherings, there are plenty of people there who are just like you—wanting to get recognized and make their own impressions. This isn't to say they are not worth talking to; however, they likely are not interested in the details of what you do. After the usual courteous formalities, you may want to move on to talk with others who may be interested about what you do.

Step 4 - Follow-up with those who express an interest

If you do arouse the interest of someone who really seems to want to know about what you do, it is time for the next step. Making a statement that shows how you can help is the first thing you want to do. "We help attorneys with those types of cases all the time," or "One of the things we do is organize the medical records which saves you a lot of time and frustration." This may be a good time to ask specific leading questions to find out more about this attorney. Eventually, ask if they would like you to send them some information or set up a brief appointment to show them examples of what you can do for them.

> **Betty's Comments:**
> Be careful not to mention any specific cases that you may have been involved with—either by name or by situation. This could be considered a breach on confidentiality—particularly if the person with whom you are speaking happens to be familiar with the case or is possibly from the opposing side!

Other occasions when you might find it necessary to "explain" yourself

You might think that the only time you need to use your 30-second introduction would be with attorney-client prospects. Nothing could be further from the truth. While that is likely the most important occasion, it isn't the only time you should be ready to use your prepared introduction. There may be occasions of chance meetings with old friends, church socials, cocktail parties, dinner parties, casual meetings on a plane/train, other organizations than those that are purely attorney-oriented. You get the picture.

If you are not talking with an attorney, your 30-second introduction does not require the leading questions. However, you still need to be as precise about what you do if you want the opportunity to explain more about your new career. You can see that you might need to prepare more than one 30-second introduction-for different occasions. After you have begun to develop and use your introduction, you will find it easier to adapt it to various occasions.

Most people are not accustomed to the name of "Legal Nurse Consultant," It sounds convoluted, and the terminology does not clearly state what you DO. If the person with whom you are talking asks what you DO, don't just

> *Most people are not accustomed to the name of "Legal Nurse Consultant*

say what you ARE (a "legal nurse consultant"). This is a more informal conversation, but it does give you the opportunity to implement what you have prepared. If the person indicates continued interest after you give your opening gambit, they will ask for clarification.

Someone might ask, "What do you do at the law firm, take blood pressures?" This is, of course, a "ha-ha" from them. Your response should be equally light-hearted. You might say, "No, I raise them!" If the conversation gets serious, it is probable the person is truly interested in learning about what you do. Now you have a chance to give a more in-depth description of what you do. You should also have that information ready in your mind at any given time. But don't bore the person to death.

Give pithy explanations of some of the specific things you can do—things this person can understand, since we are assuming they have no particular legal knowledge or medical knowledge.

It is never a waste of time to talk to people about what you do.

It is never a waste of time to talk to people about what you do. Serendipity may take over and that person may be instrumental in your getting a case or a referral. The world is wonderfully serendipitous – be ready to take advantage of it.

> **John Sez:**
> There is a fine line between someone who is always on the lookout for opportunity and someone who is a shameless self-promoter. Some of my biggest business deals have come as the result of seemingly casual conversation on airplanes and in other public places. (Notice — I scrupulously avoided saying bars.)
> If you are going to prosper as an LNC, you must always have your antenna up and be listening for opportunity. Entrepreneurs market themselves and their services on a 24/7 basis.

PRACTICE DOESN'T ALWAYS MAKE PERFECT, BUT IT DOES MAKE "PERMANENT."

You must be ready to give your 30-second introduction at any given time when you are with other people. Even your friends might want to know what it is you do, and why you call yourself a "Legal Nurse Consultant."

To be effective, you must do preparation of your statement[s] and practice it with some regularity. Not only should you write out several varied statements for your 30-

...you must do preparation of your statement[s] and practice it with regularity.

second promo and practice them, you also need to be ready to seize on an opportunity when a potential client expresses interest in your services or an acquaintance asks about what you do.

SOME FINAL TIPS

Even if someone is initially interested in what your consulting consists of, they will soon be bored if you go on and on. Pay close attention to their attention level as you talk. Curiosity may only last a

...they will soon be bored if you go on and on

few seconds to minutes. Use that time and your companion's attention with care. With practice—and practice and practice—you will get better at your 30-second introductions as well as with your leading questions. Better to leave them wanting more than to have them leave bored with you.

The Bottom Line

- ☑ Your 30-second introduction is one of your major marketing tools.
- ☑ Spend whatever time is necessary to develop, memorize, and practice your 30-second introduction.
- ☑ Only go longer in your introduction when your conversation partner shows an interest.
- ☑ Practice—practice—practice.
- ☑ Be on the lookout for opportunity, it surfaces in the strangest places.

Notes

Success is turning knowledge into positive action.
Dorothy Leeds

SECTION 10 - MASTERING THE TELEPHONE CONTACT

Our goal in this section is not to totally eliminate the butterflies, but to get them to at least fly in formation. It's OK to be nervous and have butterflies when you think about contacting strangers. It is a new marketing skill that you must learn. If you don't like talking to strangers, none of these methods are particularly pleasant.

IT ALL BEGINS WITH ATTITUDE

Our first consideration is one that most people don't think about but should. It is your attitude, or mindset, going into this process. The mind is a powerful force, and the way you think when going into a marketing call, an appointment, or a project

A positive mental attitude sets up your mind to recognize an opportunity when you see it

has a lot to do with the outcome. A positive mental attitude sets up your mind to recognize an opportunity when it occurs. A positive attitude allows you to project confidence and foster trust from your client. Being fearful of approaching strangers is natural. No one likes to risk rejection. A positive mental attitude requires constant reinforcement.

John sez:

It is important for you to understand that both direct mail and telephone contacts are designed to help you economically determine which prospects are interested in your services. Many people who start out in your pool of "prospects" will, after a mailing and a telephone contact, turn into "non-prospects."

The prospect who hangs up on you will clearly become an immediate candidate for the "no longer a prospect" category. This is not all bad, you can quit spending time and money on this person.

Other prospects will be polite, but it will be obvious that they are not really interested in your services at this time. You have to make a determination about how much time and energy you want to spend in continuing to contact this person. At this point you can decide if you want to throw them back into your pool of prospects or consider them non-prospects and quit fooling with them.

Please keep this all in perspective. Many of your initial prospects will be screened out of your prospect pool. That's what you are trying to accomplish here. You want to economically find those who are interested in your services so that you spend your marketing time and money courting the most viable prospects.

Keep in mind that this is a learning process. These are new skills and you will make some mistakes. We reiterate that marketing your services is a numbers game.

Expect a lot of people to say "no."

Expect a lot of people to say "no." This is not failure, it's feedback. Although quick jobs do occasionally happen, it often takes six months to a year after your initial contact with the potential client for a case to surface. So don't expect instant results.

Three things to remember when contacting clients.

❑ They need your service. You provide solutions for their problems.

❑ You can help them succeed in winning cases or mitigating issues.

❑ Your business is unique and interesting to most potential clients.

YOU MUST "PUSH YOURSELF"

Fear of calling holds many LNCs back. It presents quite a problem for some people and stops many from getting ahead.

Fear of calling ...stops many from getting ahead.

Since the secret of getting ahead is getting started, the first contact is your "first step on the journey." You must push yourself to change, but change is almost always painful.

Many people are so afraid of calling that they procrastinate, and they are good at the procrastination. When it comes time to call, they think of a hundred other things they would rather be doing. You may have the same problem. In order to be a successful LNC you must do whatever it takes to make those calls. Take a deep breath and dial.

Betty's comment:
Paula Woo, in her on-camera interview for Sky Lake Productions' award winning video "Profiles of Legal Nurse Consultants," told us how nervous she was before making her first telephone call. Paula said, "I threw up and then made the call and actually got a case!" Today, Paula is a highly successful LNC with an extensive client base.

BEGIN WITH THE END IN MIND

As Steven Covey teaches in his best-selling book, THE 7 HABITS OF HIGHLY EFFECTIVE PEOPLE, we want to begin with the end in mind. That is, understand what you are trying to accomplish by calling. The first thing you must do is introduce yourself (another chance to

...understand what you are trying to accomplish by calling.

use a pithy 30-second introduction). Next, you test for interest in your services. And third, you want to get a 15 to 30 minute appointment. Those are the goals. In short, the telephone call is an efficient way to see who wants to play. It's an exercise designed to separate the prospects from the non-prospects. The first preparation begins between your ears. Remember to start with a positive attitude that you can do this.

Betty's comment:
Nadine Neville-Turpin, a successful independent LNC, told me that she writes her marketing goals and posts them where she can see them. For instance, "place 5 calls per day" or "10 per week." Goal setting helps keep her focus and should help you develop and keep your focus as well. It's idea worth stealing.

HAVE YOUR APPOINTMENT BOOK OPEN

You should have your appointment book out and a pen available so that you can book the appointment. Let's face it, it would sound pretty bad if you asked for an appointment and the prospect said, "Sure, I'd like to hear about that. How about next Tuesday?" and you say, "Wait a minute, let me get my book out."

...it would sound pretty bad if you asked for an appointment and they said,... How about next Tuesday?" and you say, "Wait a minute, let me get my book out."

You should have a pad and pen ready to take notes of the conversation anyway. You will want to put these into your information file on the attorney later. Note things that a contact says that you might find useful, such as, "We do a lot of med mal work," or "We do a lot of plaintiff injury cases." It may be helpful to write down what her/his attitude was during the call. These are notes you can use for follow-up information.

Note taking helps you remember facts about the conversation for later use in calling, visiting, or writing. For instance, you document in your notes that when you last called a certain attorney, she was on her way out the door for a vacation and also was very friendly. When you contact her again you cannot only reference, "How was your vacation?" but you'll feel more at ease when you call because you know that she was friendly the last time you spoke.

Dress professionally when making calls

Next, you should dress like a professional. We know it may sound dumb, but it's a proven fact that when you look and feel successful, you project success, even over the phone. How confident and in charge can you sound wearing your bedroom shoes and housecoat? No matter what TV commercials insinuate about workers at home in their PJs and bunny slippers, you'll feel more professional in a decent outfit.

How confident and in charge can you sound wearing your bunny slippers...

Another old but useful tip is to put a mirror on your desk and smile as you dial. There is no denying that a smile comes through in your voice on the telephone.

Finally, a no-brainer. Close the door and keep distractions to a minimum. We are talking barking dogs, blaring TVs, clothes dryer buzzers, and kids here.

WHAT DO I SAY WHEN I CALL?

Now you are ready to call, but what do you say? In the situation where you actually get through to your potential client, here is one version you might consider.

> "I'm Laura Jones, a legal nurse consultant. I recently sent you some information about how I help attorneys manage their medically related cases. Do you remember receiving the information? (*If they do not remember seeing your information, start with your 30-second introduction, otherwise, start here.*)
>
> I would like to have the opportunity to personally introduce myself to you and show you some specific examples of how I can help you develop an effective strategy for your medical cases. That way, the next time a case with medical issues comes up, you will be aware of how I can help you. It will take about 15 minutes. Would this week be OK, or would sometime next week be better for you?"

It is important that you take the time to consider carefully what you are going to say. Write it down and have it in front of you. As you gain experience with it, adjust it to capture what seems to be working. Everyone has his or her own style; you must develop a script that fits yours.

> **John Sez:**
> One of the best ways I know to internalize your script is to practice it on your significant other, your friends, or anyone else that you trust to give you feedback. Rehearsing it in your mind is not the same as saying it aloud to someone else. Your goal should be to sound as if you are NOT delivering a script. You should also go for as much energy and enthusiasm as you can without sounding phony. This can only be accomplished by practice, practice, practice.

Whatever you say, do it with energy, enthusiasm, and as much confidence as you can muster. A good script delivered in a flat and impersonal tone is worse than a bad script delivered with energy and enthusiasm.

A good script delivered in a flat and impersonal tone is worse than a bad script delivered with energy and enthusiasm.

Complete your telephone contact by thanking (whoever you are talking with) for taking your call.

Fishing for additional contacts

If the prospect agrees to see you, ask, "Is there anyone else in your firm who might have an interest in what we offer?" If the answer is "yes" ask, "Would it be okay if I contacted them prior to my visit so I can meet them and tell them about my services as well?" Also ask, "Is it okay if I mention your name when I contact them?"

HOW TO HANDLE VOICE MAIL

Voice mail is everywhere and you might as well learn to work with it. On a first contact call, it is always preferable to talk with a person; this may be a "gatekeeper" (see "Working with Gatekeepers), so be

Voice mail is everywhere ... learn to work with it.

prepared. However, sometimes voice mail is all you get. To avoid leaving a message to voice mail (we don't recommend leaving voice mail messages), we suggest that you vary the times you call. If you still end up with a voice mail, then it may be used to screen calls. You might then leave a detailed message using your written statement. Ask them to call you back and be sure to speak slowly and distinctly. State your name and phone number at the beginning and at the end of the message. Personality, energy, enthusiasm, and a well-organized message will significantly increase the chances that your call will be returned.

Eight magic words for putting people at ease

Use the eight little words that set both of you at ease, "*I wonder if you could help me out?*" People like to help others. It offers a non-threatening situation and takes them from a confrontation with someone selling something to sharing their knowledge. Use of this technique will increase your chances of getting past a gatekeeper.

WORKING WITH GATEKEEPERS

Gatekeepers, as mentioned earlier, may include the receptionist, legal secretary, or paralegal for the lawyer. You need to understand that the gatekeeper's job often involves screening out undesirable interruptions for her or his employer. If you realize this, then you can approach the situation with the expectation of some resistance and not take it personally.

...your attitude toward the gatekeeper goes a long way in getting their cooperation.

Your attitude toward the gatekeeper goes a long way in getting their cooperation. Treat them with dignity and respect. Ask their name and use it often. Hearing their name gives a person a feeling of importance. Ask them for help. The point is, treat them politely and pleasantly, since they can be a real asset or a real obstacle; the choice is usually yours.

Three techniques for getting past gatekeepers

The gatekeeper will not let you by. This is rare, but you will come across this situation. Here are three techniques to help get around this situation.

1.   Call back at lunchtime. There may be another secretary on duty or you might get your prospect.

2.   Call after hours. This is usually when no one is in except the attorney. (Secretaries and paralegals are likely to go in early to work, while attorneys are more likely to stay late.)

3.   Send a letter via priority mail and hand-addressed to the prospect. In the letter, briefly describe what you can do for their firm. Explain that you have called several times, but the prospect has always been very busy. Conclude with something like, "May I make a request? I'll call Thursday, October 12th at 2:10 PM. If you are in, I would appreciate your taking my call. I promise to be brief and help you determine quickly if our services may fit your needs. If you are not in and would like to speak with me, could you have your secretary schedule a time for me to call back? Thank you for your consideration."

WHAT TO DO WHEN THE PERSON IS NOT IN

You call and the person is not in. Whenever you are told that the person is not in, or in a meeting, always ask when they (gatekeeper) would suggest that you call back. For instance, if the gatekeeper says, "Oh, around four o'clock or four thirty." You might say, "Thank you Debbie. I'll call back then at 4:20, would that be OK?" Now you have had the gatekeeper give you instructions and permission to call back at a particular time. You also made it an odd time, which helps her remember it. When you call back, state that it was requested that you call back at this time. She will likely go to greater lengths to put you through, because she told you to call back and feels more responsible—personally—for getting you through to the person you were trying to reach. If you don't happen to talk to the same person, you still have the upper hand of saying you were told to call back at this time.

> **John sez:**
> Calling is tough. Even the most experienced telephone marketers have to work at not being discouraged by telephone calling. I recognize that it takes courage to pick up that phone. You are in great danger of rejection. You will find that over a period of time you will talk to people who are absolutely delightful, those who are humor-impaired, those who are mean and grouchy, or those who are in desperately in need of a personality transplant. So what's new? You saw some of these same folks in your nursing practice, didn't you? In the clinical setting you got to deal with them face-to-face rather then on the telephone. Buck up and keep on dialing!

The Bottom Line

☑ Telephone contact begins and ends with your attitude.

☑ Push yourself. In order to be a successful LNC, you must do whatever it takes to make those calls.

☑ Develop a script in order to increase your comfort level – and practice it thoroughly.

☑ Don't forget the eight magic words: *"I wonder if you could help me out?"*

☑ Treat gatekeepers with respect, since they can help or hinder you with the lawyer.

Notes

Your customers will get better when you do.
Anonymous

SECTION 11 - MEETING WITH PROSPECTS

This section covers the ABCs of the client meeting. This is the opportunity you have been fishing for; you must be prepared in every way possible. You also want to approach this meeting with the right mindset. Think of yourself as an expert in your field. Remember you are far more knowledgeable about what you can do for the attorney. So walk in with confidence and a sincere interest in helping the prospect.

BEGIN WITH THE END IN MIND

Well, now you've done it. You have mailed your information package to your prospects, made some calls, and now someone agrees to meet with you to hear more about how you can help them. You are about to walk into a marketing interview. Are you prepared? Let's start, as with the telephone call, by beginning with the end in mind—by examining your goals.

You are about to walk into a marketing interview. Are you prepared?

Goals of Your First Meeting:
☑ Make a good first impression on the client and their staff
☑ Enable the prospect to put a name and a face together
☑ Understand the prospect's needs
☑ Begin to build trust and confidence
☑ Help the prospect understand what an LNC can do for him or her
☑ Be the one the prospect calls when the need for LNC services arises

THE MARKETING INTERVIEW

The marketing interview is different from a job interview. This is an interview in which YOU are more in charge than the prospect. After all, you asked for the meeting to make a presentation of your services. Although small talk helps break the ice (such as "What a beautiful view you have of the city here." Or "Your staff is very helpful and friendly.")—only indulge in a small amount of it. You asked for a very short time to make your presentation so get down to business. You might start with, "I realize you are busy, so let me get down to the basics." Then follow up with your prepared and practiced presentation—including your "show and tell" samples of work product.

You asked for a very short time to make your presentation so get down to business.

An important part of your presentation is to find out about the prospect's needs. The early part of your presentation should include asking several leading questions of the prospect (see the suggestions under the "30-second introduction section" for ideas). Let the prospect talk. You listen—and learn. Find out what problems the prospect has with medical cases—then show

how you can help solve those problems. If you have said you will only take 15 minutes of the prospect's time, don't take more unless they initiate the extension of time. You are not here for a "hard sell"—you want to create a good impression and let the prospect know how you can help them be more efficient and effective in their medical cases.

While you will be making your presentation, and will therefore be the speaker for a period of time, be aware that there is also power in listening. When the prospective client asks questions or makes comments, "listen" to the non-verbal as well as the verbal content. Don't let your "interview nerves" interfere with good listening. You will not be able to determine well what the potential client perceives as his problem if you do not listen well. And, if you don't understand the problems, you can't offer appropriate solutions.

Some Marketing Interview Tips:

❑ Arrive 10 to 15 minutes early. This allows you to get "settled" before the interview and also makes a good impression regarding your punctuality.

❑ Be appropriately dressed in something which feels (physically) comfortable and which increases your confidence. A skirt suit is best.

❑ Stand straight; sit straight. Your posture says a lot about you.

❑ Make eye contact and have a firm handshake. You have about three seconds in which to make your impression—use it well. This takes preparation ahead of time and rarely involves anything you have to *say* at the very beginning.

> Betty's comment:
> Remember, before any interview, a thorough knowledge of any potential client is a must. Review the information you have on this prospect before you go.

THE FIRST MEETING SETS THE TONE FOR THE FUTURE RELATIONSHIP

The first meeting is an excellent time to establish a base or character for the entire relationship between you and the prospect. Skillfully setting a positive tone is not that difficult. The secret is a basic law of human nature; people tend to respond strongly in kind to the behavior of other people. This first meeting is the best time to set your relationship into motion, because the tone and the spirit of the start is usually the tone and the spirit of the entire relationship.

...people tend to respond strongly in kind to the behavior of other people.

MAKE A GOOD FIRST IMPRESSION

Several business books on making a good impression, state that you have only a few seconds—yes, seconds—to make your first impression. Most of it comes through in your non-verbal communication. This starts, as we have already noted, with how your confidence—through your prepared mindset—comes through, as well as how you are dressed. (See *Section 15: Establishing Your Credibility* for more details.) Your walk, poise, smile, and eye contact deliver this impression. When you set your expectation ahead of time to believe you have something worth while to offer this prospect, this can come through in your first few seconds as well. Enthusiasm, energy, and sincerity should be a part of your mindset; don't let that appear to be arrogance or a salesman's overstatement though. Also remember that sometimes you make first impressions on the staff even before you meet the "boss."

Okay, we all agree that a first impression is a lasting one. There are some other tricks to help you get through this first meeting more successfully. Always arrive a few minutes early. If you arrive late, no matter what the excuse, you are immediately pitching from behind.

Arriving early allows you the opportunity to get your thoughts together and to meet the gatekeeper(s). Make sure to get the gatekeeper's name and, if the opportunity presents itself, have a brief conversation. (If you have been keeping good notes you should already know some names because of prior telephone contacts.)

Wouldn't you rather have them say "she was very nice" than to say, "Who was that bozo?"

Let them do most of the talking. This is great practice for the meeting coming up. Try to leave them with a positive feeling about you. You might be surprised at the comments the secretary, and others, may have about you to the boss after you leave. Wouldn't you rather have them say "she was very nice" than to say, "Who was that bozo?" Make them feel important. Ignoring them or treating them like a second class citizen is the best way to get the "bozo" comment and a bad attitude every time you call back.

As an aside, don't let your nervousness be interpreted as being aloof or arrogant. You may have no intention of treating anyone badly, but your own nervousness may make you appear that way. Use the old

...don't let your nervousness be interpreted as being aloof or arrogant.

technique of pretending you are welcoming someone into YOUR home. You are the hostess.

Consider it your responsibility to make them comfortable. It is probable they want to make you comfortable as well. You didn't get this interview because they wanted to annoy you. If you have gotten this far with a prospect, he is interested in what you have to say.

John Sez.
Part of being able to pull this off is looking and feeling as professional as possible. Wear the absolute best suit, shoes, and matching accessories that you can afford. You will be amazed at the boost in self-confidence that dressing professionally gives you. Beside that, it makes you look like you are worth what you charge.

Betty's comment:
Let's get down to the nitty-gritty. The whole package counts. The details of grooming and accessories are noticed and can significantly affect that critical first impression. Wear a new pair of hose so you will know there are no runs or snags to worry about. And , as for shoes, make sure they are not scuffed or dirty. Men particularly notice shoes and women are likely to notice bad hosiery. Also, wear your prettiest lingerie underneath. While these won't be "noticed," it will make you feel special and more comfortable "in your skin."

THE POWER OF A SMILE

People expert, Les Giblin, in his book HOW TO BE PEOPLE SMART, says "In the first second, that instant when you establish eye contact before you say anything, give people your <u>sincere</u> smile. The result, they

Remember to smile before you break the silence.

will smile back. This is the surest, fastest, easiest way for you to win people over." This simple technique is a must with experts and should be a must for you. Remember to smile before you break the silence, before you say "hello," "good morning," or anything else. A smile before you say anything is much more effective than at any other time. Try it in different situations for a week and see for yourself—in the grocery line, at the bank teller, in a retail store. You will be astonished at how people will react to you. Above all, be sincere. People in general, and women in particular, can spot a phony smile from a mile away. Don't even think about trying to fake it.

Betty's Comment:
There is an added dividend to practicing your smiling approach in various situations. That dividend is that YOU will feel the effects of the smile internally and are very likely to begin to be truly more friendly and open to people. This can reduce stress and actually change your whole attitude — if you have any of the "people are rude and uncaring" belief. Become aware of your behavior in as many situations as you can. You may be projecting an attitude that you do not intend. Putting a smile on your face is an obligation to put a smile on your behavior as well.

QUESTIONS THAT ARE DESIGNED TO UNCOVER NEEDS

Along with the information you have already gleaned by researching this firm/attorney in Martindale-Hubbell or other sources, you also need to have notes on some of the questions you plan to ask. <u>Write questions out in advance</u> and glance at them as you go through the interview. You should be taking notes of the answers as well. It is perfectly appropriate to take notes of this meeting. In fact, we have included a form for this purpose in Appendix B.

You should be taking notes of the answers as well.

Adapt this form for your personal use. Your prospect should appreciate your organization and attention to noting what his problems include. As in your 30-second introduction, be prepared to ask leading questions that will tell you about the prospect's perceived needs. (Note that the prospect may perceive his needs differently than you.)

> **John Sez:**
> Write questions in advance. Do not try to wing it. I am never embarrassed to say to a client "excuse me a minute while I check my notes and make sure that I have asked you everything I intended to."

Here are a few examples:

"Tell me about your practice in regard to medical issues." Try to get a good feel for the type of practice they have beyond what you have already learned by research. You should already have confirmed the fact that you know something about what this attorney does, e.g. medical malpractice, products liability; however, you can note that you would like to know some of the client's specific problems that crop up in cases with medical issues.

Another question might be, "What areas do you particularly specialize in?" Remember, people like to feel important. You make them feel important by asking about their work, listening to them, using their name often, and complimenting them—appropriately.

Other appropriate questions are some of the same ones you might have prepared for your follow-up information of your 30-second introduction. "Who do you usually depend upon for your medical records organization and analysis?" "What has your experience been with Legal Nurse Consultants?"

...listen to what is being said between the lines.

Take notes of anything that may be helpful later. Take notes and listen to what is being said between the lines.

Another tip is to pause slightly before answering a question posed by the prospect. You increase the other person's trust by letting them know that their question is important. You flatter them by giving them the courtesy of taking time to consider their question. You might respond with, "That's a good question" (if indeed it is). It gives them a compliment and you a break to form the proper response. Lean toward the person with interest and look at them when they are speaking.

Betty's Comment:
Listening is a learned skill. You should have good practice in this already, since you have been taught to listen to your patients. However, you will be in a different setting in the law firm and will have a different set of stressors. Practice listening with your family and friends. Test your ability to listen by summarizing and repeating back to a family member or friend what they have just said. Then ask them if you got it right. This is called "testing for understanding." It is a good technique to use with a client—summarize and repeat back to be sure that you have clearly understood them. If you practice good listening techniques, it will be one less thing you have to worry about when you go on a marketing interview,.

DETERMINE WHERE THIS PERSON FITS ON THE "HIERARCHY OF PROSPECTS"

Based on what you learn from listening, you will need to transition from listening to helping the prospect understand what LNCs do and how you, specifically, might help them solve their problems. This is the teaching part. If your prospect is from the "Unaware" category, you may have to start with teaching them the basics of what LNCs can do for clients. This is a good time to review your brochure with them and elaborate on the items that seem to fit their needs. If they are from the "Aware but Unconvinced" category, you should approach your "teaching" on a slightly different basis. Your questioning should have uncovered the areas in which they are unconvinced. Don't argue with the prospect; present positive approaches to the issues about which they are unconvinced.

WHY WORK PRODUCT SAMPLES ARE A KILLER MARKETING TOOL

Your work product samples are a key to helping prospects understand what you can do for them. And isn't this the reason for your visit to them?

If the prospect is from the Aware but Unconvinced or Hot Prospect category, you will need to build confidence and trust in order to get their business. In short, you need to look and act as if you know what you are doing (even if you feel a bit overwhelmed). This is where "never let them see you sweat" applies. You can spend less time "telling" and more time showing them examples of your work product. They need to understand what you can do for them; work product is the best tool that you have to develop that understanding. Work product samples provide actual, real examples of what you can do to help them in presenting their cases.

Work product samples are one of the most important sales tools the LNC has available.

As referred to earlier, always disguise the case names. Your "sample" should never give a clue about the patient, the doctor(s), or the hospital from which the records came. Breach of confidence is still a concern when you show a sample of work. Don't risk appearing as a novice who is unaware of the importance of confidentiality.

> **Betty's Comment:**
> It could happen that the lawyer/prospect knows the case or the attorneys in the case that you are using for your example—even when you attempt to disguise the case. They might think they can "pick your brain" for clues about how that attorney (whom you worked with) thinks. Don't get sucked into discussion on the case itself beyond presenting how you developed the work product or located the supporting research.

A CAUTION ABOUT WORK PRODUCT SAMPLES

Occasionally a potential client will ask for copies of your work product samples. In some cases, they might have in mind using these as teaching examples for their current staff. You will have to make a decision about sharing this information. As a general rule, we do NOT recommend that you leave behind copies of your samples. What you need to make clear is that the

...we do NOT recommend that you leave behind copies of your samples.

format of the samples is not nearly as important as your analysis and clarification of the medical issues involved. Having a paralegal use your format to summarize records is not the same as having you do assessment and research of the issues. You obviously have an advantage over a paralegal—even if she has been doing this summarizing for years. However, you should never imply that a paralegal was not doing a good job. Your approach is to point out the added value of your work product in regard to medical issues. Never denigrate anyone else to put yourself forward; that includes doctors as well as paralegals or other nurses.

HOLD OFF ON GIVING ADVICE

During the first interview, many new LNCs are so eager to help the potential client and show that they recognize the problem and the solution, that they begin giving advice on a case described by the attorney. Here are two reasons to avoid doing that: (1) In almost every situation you will not yet know enough about the case to give sound advice; (2) sometimes a potential client will take your advice but use their existing staff to implement it.

...do not volunteer anything until you have negotiated ... involvement for yourself.

You can let the prospect know that you are familiar with that disease process or issue but state that you would hesitate to offer any suggestions without reviewing ALL the records. Offer to read the records and give your comments at a later time. Even if the solution seems perfectly clear to you, do not volunteer anything until you have negotiated some involvement for yourself. If you solve the prospect's perceived problem, why should he hire you?

Betty's Comments:
Never make judgments on what you are TOLD by the attorney or his client; they often have misunderstood or unintentionally mischaracterized the facts or situation. Your job is always to review ALL the records before making assessments on the factual issues. A review of the records may show a different situation altogether. I speak from personal experience—with egg on my face to prove it.

YOU WANT TO BE REMEMBERED

We presented this scenario before but it bears repeating:

"She arrives, professionally dressed, with a box of goodies for the office (donuts, granola bars, flowers, etc.). She takes the time to meet the receptionist and the secretaries. She meets with the potential client; listens to his problems; shows him some of her work samples that are relevant to the client's problems; goes over her brochure to help them understand the services she offers and how those services can give the client an edge over their opponents in the case. She leaves them with several copies of her brochure, business card, and Rolodex® card (one to keep, one to share). At the end of the interview, she asks the potential client, "Who else do you know that needs to hear about my services?" A day after the interview she sends them a follow-up note thanking them for sharing their time with her." Following this approach format, you should have results from your visits with potential clients.

THE POWER OF GOODIES

We have spoken of "goodies" several times. Doughnuts, candy, granola bars, fruit, or flowers always are appreciated and can go a long way in helping you be remembered. Gatekeepers will particularly appreciate your thinking of them in this way. Providing small pleasures for them helps

Don't overlook this powerful and inexpensive way to differentiate yourself.

break up an office day and will help them remember you. Try to find out the size of the office and take some doughnuts or cookies with you. Otherwise, you might plan to send something later-whether that day or the following. Keep in mind that what you send should include the whole office if it is a small one or should be of sufficient quantity to share with at least a good sized group if the office is larger. Don't overlook this powerful and inexpensive way to differentiate yourself.

A respected colleague of ours purchases a small, tasteful (and tasty) box of assorted goodies at an upper-class bakery in Atlanta. She affixes a small gold seal, which she has had printed for her use, on it that says, "compliments of PSA Medical Legal Consulting."

The method you choose to use and the type of goodies you select are a personal decision on your part. Home made or professionally prepared, it really doesn't matter. What does matter is that goodies have excellent marketing power. This approach indicates good social manners and thoughtfulness in an acceptable way. You can give yourself a competitive edge over someone who doesn't use them.

John Sez:
The debate rages in our household on the issue of home made vs. store bought. Some LNCs have stated, in no uncertain terms, that they believe home made is "unprofessional." On the other hand, one of my graduate students (MBA) went from selling $100,000 a year in textbooks (she worked for a book publisher) to over a million a year in just three years. Basically she developed relationships with her clients by using her home baked chocolate chip cookies as a way to differentiate herself from her competitors. She has had to hire three little old ladies to bake for her, because she no longer has the time.

HOW TO AVOID THE MISTAKE MADE BY MANY LNCs

One of the major problems with new and inexperienced LNCs is that they frequently fail to ask for the prospect's business. Do not be guilty of this fundamental error. ASK FOR THEIR BUSINESS. If you don't ask, you will never

If you don't ask (for their business), you will never know what opportunity was missed.

know what opportunity was missed. Do not be shy or obtuse about it; simply say " I would like to work with you in the future and would appreciate an opportunity to show you what I can do to help you. I think you will be pleased with the results."

> **Betty's comment:**
> If you don't ask, you may never get. Don't be bashful — you're in a new professional arena , namely, the business world.

THINGS YOU NEED TO CONSIDER WHEN NEGOTIATING FOR YOUR FIRST WORK FROM A PROSPECT

If you have discovered that the prospect has a current case with which you could help, offer to do so. If you have listened well, you should have a good "feel" for what the prospect needs and how they might respond. It is likely that they do have a need for help in a medical case, since most lawyers do not spend time with people marketing themselves if they don't see a current need for the marketer. The lawyer's time is too valuable (they get paid for their own "billable" hours) to spend interviewing you just because you asked.

Don't offer to work for free but do offer a "special opportunity"

Negotiating should always be a win-win situation.

for the prospect to see what you can do to help in medically related cases. Negotiating should always be a win-win situation. Give the client a good deal but make your value clear as well.

Do not simply offer to do the work for a cheap price. Be very

be clear with yourself about what you charge BEFORE you do any marketing

specific about what your rate is (and you should always be clear with yourself about what you charge BEFORE you do any marketing), but say you will do the case for "X" amount per hour instead. That lets the prospect know that you feel sure enough about your value to do a "test" case. If you don't state up front what your "regular" rate is for work, you may be stuck doing work for this client at a very low rate. You might then have a difficult time raising this to your regular rate in the future.

If you detect hesitancy at your first offer, you might suggest you could review the records and give a narrative report—or prepare a time line about an issue the prospect has referred to—for a specified flat rate in the case. In other words, "I would be willing to review the records and do a time line of the medications this person took (if that is important to the case) for a flat rate of $375." However, you must again be specific about what you will do for that flat rate offer.

You need to have some idea as to the amount of records that need reviewing before you come up with a flat rate—and you should make it clear you are offering a discounted rate. Even if you "lose" money because it takes you longer than you thought, you have the opportunity to show what you can do to help, and the client knows exactly what it will cost. This is a winner for the client and a winner for you as well. You have a chance to get a new client—which is what you want—and the client gets a thorough job done on his medical issues.

> **Betty's comment:**
> When you bill the client for work that you negotiated at a discount, always show your regular fees for the work — then show the discount as a reduction from your regular rate.

Negotiating requires flexibility on both sides. The goal is to have a good outcome for all involved. Both sides have specific needs and expectations. Being aware that your own expectations and needs are not the same as the prospect's is basic to understanding the process of negotiating. You must be prepared with ideas of how you might request work and be willing to negotiate that process so that you both come away with a feeling of satisfaction.

Once negotiation is complete, make sure you are clear about what is expected of you. It is also smart to get a portion of the anticipated charges—up front. You can take notes about what is wanted while in the interview and send a copy of the contract the next day. Tell the new client that you will provide a contract for him to sign and return to you and a copy for the client to keep as well (See the example of a simple contract in appendix B.)

Betty's comment:
Having a simple contract for your services is important. Particularly with a new client, it sets everything out clearly. State all that you have requested to do and state the fee to be charged. Make clear that the rate is discounted (if it is).

ANOTHER WAY TO BE REMEMBERED WELL

The day of the interview with the prospect, write a letter thanking them for the time allowed you. Certainly, send this no later than the following day. This thoughtfulness on your part may be what sets you apart from others with whom they may have talked. Even if they haven't talked with others, this gives you a chance to make another contact with them—which sets you up in their mind as the person to call when they need a nurse consultant.

If you have negotiated some work from them, be sure to send the contract letter—two copies—one for them to sign and return to you and one for them to keep. This is a business-like way to do business.

The Bottom Line

☑ Arrive early and well-prepared.

☑ Use your three seconds well to make a good impression.

☑ Dress professionally and smile.

☑ Consider using goodies as a marketing tool.

☑ The first meeting sets the tone for the future relationship.

☑ Leading questions will get you the information you require to understand the prospect's perceived needs.

☑ Ask for their business and be ready to negotiate an opportunity.

☑ Negotiation should be a win-win situation.

☑ Always send a thank-you note in follow up— stat.

☑ If work was negotiated, send a simple contract setting out what was requested, for what price, and when it is due.

Opportunities are usually disguised as hard work,
so most people don't recognize them.
Ann Landers

SECTION 12 - NETWORKING AS A MARKETING STRATEGY

There is an adage that says "the opposite of networking is *not-working.*" This may be very close to the truth. Networks and networking are treated as two different topics in this section. Both are important.

WHAT IS A "NETWORK?"

Too often people think of networking only in terms of going out to meet strangers and handing out business cards. This is true only to a point. There is more than one way to "network."

There is more than one way to "network."

As you join organizations that relate to your career, you are developing a network. As you get to know others who do the same or similar work as you, you are developing a network. As you get to know more clients or potential clients, you are developing a network.

So what is a network? It assuredly is more than a group of strangers for whom you must gather up your courage to meet. It is also more than a "gossip" group. A network is a group of people with similar interests and knowledge with whom you have, or will develop, a relationship. The relationship will vary.

With some you will know them only as acquaintances that have a similar interest as you. Others will be closer relationships, as in members of a common organization—such as the local and national chapters of the American Association of Legal Nurse Consultants. Or they may be a member of an online listserv that has an interest in or an association with legal nurse consulting. Clients, or potential clients, with whom you keep in contact are part of your network also.

You may have several "networks" on which you rely: A professional network, a referral network, a peer network, a lay-person network. Some are self-

You may have several "networks" on which you rely...

explanatory and some of these may be combined; don't leave out people simply because they don't fit into your professional or referral network. A lay network, which here means people who are associated with neither legal nor medical issues, is still a good source of support and stability for you. They can also be surprisingly helpful in referrals in some situations. The people in your lay network might include your spouse, a good friend who has marketing or secretarial experience, social contacts who have "connections," and people who just make you feel good by being around them.

However, a network is not simply knowing others in the same field. It is a give-and-take situation for all concerned. A

...a network is not just knowing others in the same field...

definition of a network, that you will not necessarily find in a dictionary, is that it is an informal group of people who have interrelated interests and who offer support, encouragement, and actual help to each other on various occasions or in various situations. "Network" is also used as a verb form and, as such, could be defined as, "the process of mutually offered help, support, and encouragement in an informal group that has interests that are similar." Therefore, we could combine the two forms of network by saying it is a group that involves action and reaction.

NOURISH YOUR NETWORK

A network needs to be nourished. That means, "networking your network" by keeping in contact—especially when you don't want anything from them. Let them know through your actions that you are dependable and can be trusted. They may have a need—or a referral—for someone like you in the future. They should think of you if you have done your networking correctly.

Keep confidences that you have *Don't gossip or complain* been privy to among your *about others, ever!!.* network. Don't gossip or complain about others, ever! Send out special pieces of information that designated participants may find useful—such as news articles that they may have an interest in or information about an upcoming seminar or meeting. Or just send them a joke (not off-color or mean) to bring a smile to them. Try to give as good as you receive—understanding that this is a choice and not a "should."

We are not suggesting that you go "overboard" and constantly feed your network. This can be an irritation as much as being seen as helpful. You might be seen as someone who is always sending items for which the recipient eventually feels they "owe" you rather than having them feel they want to respond in kind. This brings one to consider the adage, "you scratch my back and I'll scratch yours." That might be appropriate; however, doing something for someone in your network should not be for the consideration that they will "owe" you. You do reap what you sow—for good or ill—but that should not be the reason for offering help or support to someone. A genuine concern for and interest in others will provide you more satisfaction and, eventually, more genuine response from others as well.

ADDING TO YOUR NETWORK

You may think that the larger your network the better. Maybe. A network should be no larger than you can relate to in an effective way. It is realistic that you will be in contact with some of your network only on an occasional basis. This is appropriate and expected by most people with whom you network.

> *A network should be no larger than you can relate to...(effectively).*

But do keep in mind that everyone in your network needs an occasional contact if you plan to continue the relationship. Adding people to your special network(s) means that you take responsibility for maintaining a supportive interrelationship on at least an occasional basis. A network is dynamic, having its own pattern of growth and change. You will need to add people to your network to keep it fresh and growing. You will also lose some people over time.

> **Betty's comment:**
> Try to find yourself a mentor — an LNC with experience who is willing to be available and helpful to you. Later, as you become more experienced, mentor someone else. It's the old nursing counterpart to "see one, do one, teach one." This helps develop your network in the best way.

NETWORKING AT A LARGE GROUP GATHERING

When people talk about networking, they usually think in terms of getting dressed in their business best (and you should) and going out to "impress" folks they want to get work from in the future—or continue to get work from in other situations. Absolutely. That is a major facet of networking. The group may be a Chamber of Commerce affair, a bar association meeting, a cocktail party of business or law firms. There are many situations in which to network. Wherever you go, you are representing your personal self as well as your business self. As an independent practitioner, this line blurs; some people don't distinguish between them, which means that you usually represent both "entities" at the same time.

Five large-group networking tips and techniques that will bring results.

Tip 1: Wear comfortable but professional clothing

As we have referred to previously, wear professional looking clothes—which are comfortable. We also suggest that women wear professional looking but comfortable shoes. Spike heels may look sexy, but are they comfortable? Is sexy the look you are going for? (It shouldn't be.) However, do wear clothes and shoes in which you feel you look attractive and professional. This can help you feel good about yourself and not have to be concerned with a tight or uncomfortable outfit.

It is a good idea to wear something that has pockets in which you can place a click pen and your business cards. For women, don't carry a purse so full of items you can't find what you want—in case you need more business cards or other information while you are talking to someone. You will need both hands free at most gatherings—to hold food or drinks and to hand out your cards as appropriate. When going to a large gathering, take everything out of your purse that you do not need for the gathering. Even better, take a much smaller purse than your usual carry-all.

Tip 2: Moving around

When you are at this type of gathering/seminar/meeting/ cocktail party, you need to keep moving around to meet different people. If you do find some "soul mate" with interests like yours, you may wish to move around together—for support and courage However, there are times you need to meet as many people as "politely" possible on your own. Politeness in meeting people means you show an interest in them without trying to hard sell yourself. You need to allow enough time per meeting each person to make them feel you are talking with them because you find them interesting. Other people are here for the same reason you are. Use your 30-second introduction technique to gauge their interest in you as well as to tell about yourself. Quality encounters count for more than the quantity.

Tip 3: Escaping someone who is monopolizing your time

On occasion, when you have joined up with or been joined by someone, as mentioned above, you may have trouble escaping them if you wish to go it alone. You can plan an escape in several different ways. You can suggest you are monopolizing them, and that you both should move on to talk with other people. Or you can join a group and, after introducing your companion/monopolizer, leave the group without him/her tagging along. You may also try the ruse that you see someone across the room that you must speak with and simply excuse yourself and walk away. Do try to be polite when trying to disconnect from a monopolizer. This person could end up being a good network member for you in the future.

Tip 4: Breaking the ice at a gathering

How do you get started talking with someone or a group? One way is to pretend you are the host of the party and that it is your responsibility to see that others are comfortable. Accept that you won't be the only person there who feels uncomfortable. If you see someone alone, talk to them for a few minutes and find out about them. Ask how they happen to be at this gathering, where they came from, do they like the food? Keep the conversation light and the attention on them. This is an opportunity to practice your socializing skills.

Make eye contact with the person. You will probably not shake hands—most don't at these type of gatherings (you have too much for your hands to do already). However, if someone offers to shake your hand, be sure you have a firm, responsive grip.

Again, the two of you may join up for a few minutes to get you both into the conversation of a group. Continue the role of the host and be ready to point out some interest or an experience of your new acquaintance to a group. Make sure you are comfortable with the etiquette of introductions before you go to a meeting of this type. Introducing someone can be an uncomfortable situation if you don't know the appropriate etiquette and feel awkward doing it.

To join a group, you might stand on the fringes of the group and listen to their conversation—without interrupting them— and determine if you want to join the group. On occasion, someone in the group will offer you an entree into their conversation. Be gracious and don't take over the whole conversation. Listen to yourself—would you want to be on the receiving end of your conversation?

Keep a pleasant look on your face when with a group or standing alone. This may make it easier for other people to approach you and talk with you. A "pleasant look" doesn't necessarily mean a big smile. People may wonder what you are smiling at, "like a Cheshire cat." Just keep pleasant thoughts in your mind as you move around or join a group. Go with the mindset that people are going to like you—why shouldn't they? Your features will show your pleasant state of mind. An interesting quote by André Dubus keeps me grounded: "Shyness has a strange element of narcissism, a belief that how we look, how we perform, is truly important to other people."

Tip 5: Use your business cards well

You don't have to give a card to every person you speak with. It should arise naturally in your conversation as you both talk (be sure you have practiced your 30-second introduction). If you want to give the other person your card, but they haven't asked for it, ask for their card. They may then request yours in return; at least you can offer yours more readily. Be sure you have plenty of business cards but put only a few at a time in your pocket or business card holder—you don't want it to appear you have brought enough for the "whole world." They should feel special that you are interested in them and want their card.

You should also have a click pen in your pocket. You want to be able to use the pen to write using only one hand, rather than needing an additional hand (and not your teeth, please) to take the cap off a pen or have to twist it to get the point down. Remember, you are likely to be holding a drink at the least. Why a pen at all? Because when you receive business cards from another, you may want to write down some additional information they give you. At the least, as soon as you walk away you should make a note about them that reminds you of what you talked about or something special about them. You may have use for this information later. This will be a good reference if you decide to write them a note in follow-up. Referring to a specific topic discussed with them (and identifying the meeting place and time) may help them recall who you are—and may impress them with your attentiveness.

LARGE GROUP NETWORKING CAVEATS

When you are at a cocktail party or other type of large group gathering, there are several things to keep in mind:

❑   The first and foremost is not to drink too much—get a glass of club soda or water with a piece of lemon and stick with it. Having a drink (of water preferably) in your hand is not only acceptable but is the expected at a cocktail party. However, there is nothing that ruins your impression more than the appearance of having had too much alcohol.

❑   Don't eat too much. You did not come for the food—although it may be very good. If you want to eat some of the hors d'oeuvres, do so at the beginning and eat all at once so you will be free to move around and use your hands as you talk with people. You can also go to the hors d'oeuvre table to look as if you have something to do when you really don't know what to do next. Talk to anyone else there—about the food. Then move on again.

❑   Don't gossip about or make fun of other people—they may be friends or significant others of the person with whom you are talking. Besides that, it's just plain tacky.

❑   Don't talk about your problems and woes. It is a party—or at least a cordial gathering. Be upbeat in your conversation; it will make you feel better too.

❑   Don't talk politics or religion. Enough said!!!

The Bottom Line

☑ A "network" is a group of people with whom you have developed a relationship.

☑ Networking involves as much "give" as "take."

☑ Don't hard sell yourself to your networks or while networking.

☑ Networking in a large group gathering requires social skills such as the etiquette of introductions.

☑ Make notes about the people from whom you get business cards—on the back of their card.

☑ In large group gatherings, DON'T – drink too much, eat too much, gossip (at all), or talk about religion or politics.

There's no traffic jam on the extra mile.
Anonymous

SECTION 13 - REFERRALS AS A MARKETING STRATEGY

Referrals should become a major source of clients and new business as you become established. As you build your client base, you will be spending less time on direct mail and cold-calling activities. Much of your new business should be coming from referrals.

WHAT EVERY LNC NEEDS TO KNOW ABOUT ASKING FOR REFERRALS

Referrals are a major generator of business in the legal world. Lawyers make and receive referrals all the time, consequently they understand, and are comfortable with, the referral process.

Be sure to ask your satisfied clients for referrals. Get the names of two or three other persons who need your services. When a

Be sure to ask your satisfied clients for referrals.

client gives you a name, ask for additional information about the referral prospect. Based on that information, you can decide if this is a prospect worth pursuing. Also, be sure that the referring attorney will allow you to use his name as having referred you.

Most truly satisfied clients will be delighted to give you referrals and a significant number of these referrals will become a client. Ask if you may use your current client's name when making contact with the referral.

Sometimes the referral will come to you without your having contacted them. This may happen when a satisfied client gives your name to another lawyer and suggests he call you to help with a medical case. However, it is not as likely to happen as when you ask for referrals.

John Sez:
Once again the ball is in your court, take it and run.

HOW TO TURN YOUR CLIENTS INTO GOODWILL AMBASSADORS

Ask for testimonial letters

Most satisfied clients don't tell others about your great work unless you ask them to. Each time you have a satisfied client, ask them to write a letter, on their letterhead stationary, stating how pleased they were with your services. If your client doesn't know what to say, show them copies of others letters or compose a sample letter for them. Given a model, most clients will have no trouble writing a great testimonial in their own words.

Ask for these testimonial letters when you are checking with the client to see if they are happy with your work. You need to do this on a regular basis anyway.

Testimonial letters can be included in your portfolio of information when you visit a new prospect. We don't suggest you mail out copies of them willy-nilly. However, if you are writing a letter to someone specifically referred to you by a client, you might include a copy of the letter from your client. Note we said a copy; you keep the original in your file.

One last thing, when a client does give you a referral or a testimonial letter, thank him. Send a thank-you note or send a small tasty gift (as previously suggested under "goodies"). If given the opportunity, consider taking the client out to lunch (of course, YOU pay).

> **Betty's comment:**
> Again, if you don't ask—you won't get. It is necessary that you know that your client actually is happy with your work.

Ask if you can use them as a future reference

Be sure to ask your clients if you can use them as references for

...ask your clients if you can use them as references...

your future clients or marketing. This can be a valuable addition to your brochure. Having the names of several high-profile attorneys and their firms as references (or clients) is a big credibility builder. Ask for this even if they have no names to give you as a referral. You want to be sure it is okay to use their name in a letter or in a brochure.

HOW TO MAKE REFERRALS A WIN-WIN SITUATION

You can give your current client even more incentive to provide names for referrals if you offer them something in return. Consider giving them a discount on a future case or a "certificate" for "x" number of hours of work on a future case for every person they refer that actually gives you a case. The attorney may even be more likely to "talk you up" to another attorney for that possible benefit. Your attorney client has now become a part of your professional or referral network. Keep this client supplied with small bits of information for cases that you know he has. This keeps your name fresh in his mind. Go that extra mile for your current client—do more than is expected. Provide excellent value for your fees. This is the kind of behavior that can get you referrals—IF you learn to ask for them.

Although mentioned previously, it is always important to ask if there are other attorneys in the same firm that might be able to use your services. This is an area of referral that is surprisingly overlooked by the LNC. Some firms do personal injury as well as medical malpractice cases, and your services can be of benefit to both types. Products liability cases are another type in which you can offer great help. Make it clear that you can be of value in more than just medical malpractice work. Also, make clear that you can identify and locate expert witnesses or provide research on the opposing side's expert. You may need to continually provide education to your attorney-client about all the benefits you can provide as an LNC.

... it is always important to ask if there are other attorneys in the same firm that might be able to use your services...

ASK OTHERS BESIDES LAWYERS FOR REFERRALS

Other sources of referrals are your friends, people you know socially, fellow church members, etc. Do not be shy about asking, "who do you know that might need my services?" Again, the same rules apply as when asking your clients, that is, ask if you can use their name and ask them why they think that person needs your service. This is an example of your lay person network. This person deserves thanks and continued

Do not be shy about asking, "who do you know that might need my services?"

consideration from you also—a thank-you note or a small gift for a good reference. Don't abuse your relationship with your friends and acquaintances. Their main responsibility is to be your friend or acquaintance—not your public relations firm.

The Bottom Line

☑ Over time, referrals should become a major source of new clients.

☑ Attorneys understand and support the referral process. That is often how they get new business.

☑ Always ask for referrals – even within the same firm.

☑ If you sense that a client is very pleased with your work, ask for a testimonial letter.

☑ Make referrals a win-win situation.

☑ Friends and others can be an excellent source of referrals.

Everyone is trying to accomplish something big,
not realizing that life is made up of little things.
Frank A. Clark

SECTION 14– OTHER LOW-
COST MARKETING STRATEGIES

Your major marketing strategies will be those methods we have
already discussed; however, there are other ways to market that
you can use to boost your overall strategies. This Section offers
some additional ways to do this.

DOING CASES FOR LITTLE OR NOTHING

Pro Bono work

Pro bono means to do work for free—for the good of those
who cannot afford it. Doing pro bono work with a lawyer or
firm can be a way for you to build up your skills and get
experience. Every law firm is expected to do pro bono work to
some extent. The trick is to be certain that the case you are
working on is actually a pro bono case—not just a case they want
you to do for free.

Legal Aid Society

Check your phone book for the local legal aid society. Legal aid often is done at a very low cost to the clients. The legal aid group might need your services in some cases but would not be able (or willing) to pay very much. However, working with them increases your network of lawyers that you know and gives you valuable experience.

SPEAKING AND WRITING

Whether you decide to present yourself in writing or speaking venues or both, you must be knowledgeable about legal nurse consulting. You may have the skills to write and speak, and you may have the medical and nursing knowledge to offer, but you must also know what is of value in this combination for the lawyers who attend the meeting or read the article. Both these activities are opportunities to add to your network of informed lawyers who may become prospects or clients of yours.

You might offer to speak to your local bar association group about a medical issue that is of interest to them; this would put you in the position of being presented as the knowledgeable person to whom they can refer. Be sure to take your brochures and business cards along with any other appropriate marketing materials, but don't make this a "hard sell" meeting. You are there to present "medical" information and to impress them with your knowledge that would be of help to them in any medical issue case.

You are there to present "medical" information and to impress them...

A caveat to speaking to groups: If you are asked specific questions about a case, don't try to "solve" it there. This is the same concept as your offering solutions to a case when your are just visiting for an interview. You may be giving away the store and get little or nothing in return. Remember your marketing visit to an attorney's office – respond that it sounds interesting but that you would need to see all the medical records before you could make an assessment of the situation. You can offer an hour's free evaluation or some other incentive to get the business, but at least, expect something in return.

Another idea that might be used when invited to speak—specifically to a group of lawyers—is to have a "prize" drawing. Have each lawyer put his or her card in a bowl and have a drawing at the end of the speech. The *have a "prize" drawing* winner can be given a specified number of hours of free work or use the "buy one get one" idea of doing a free case evaluation when they send you one for pay. Whatever you decide, of course, can be the prize. Just remember that both of you should "win" something.

Don't overlook the opportunity to speak to groups that are comprised of all types of business people–such as the Lion's Club, Kiwanis, Chamber of Commerce, or others. At a meeting like this, you would present medical information as well. Make it about something the whole group might have an interest in such as a new medical technique, or new drugs, or some current health concern of the community. This would mean that you would have the topic well-researched and even offer references–for both library and Internet.

Writing articles can also be a good marketing strategy. Again, you must be knowledgeable about legal nurse consulting as well as your specific topic—which might be information about Medicaid, Workers Compensation, ERISA, HMOs, etc. Be sure you research your topic and present an unbiased, well-documented article. This is not everyone's forte. Only do this if you feel comfortable about your writing skills. One place to have your article printed is in the newsletter (if they have one) of your local bar association.

Not surprisingly, there is a caveat about this as well. Be careful that your article is balanced regarding plaintiff and defense issues–UNLESS you are doing it for a plaintiff group or for a defense group. Some LNCs never seem to realize there is "another side" to the issue–except they may be inclined to denigrate the other side in general. Even IF writing an article for a specific plaintiff or defense group, you should keep a balanced, unbiased approach. Your integrity is what is at stake, not what "they want to hear."

Betty's Comment:
Do not approach the article from a "legal" standpoint. You are not the lawyer—they are. However, you can tie the legal viewpoints of others to the medical concepts. For example, if you were writing an article titled, "How to assess your client's medical records for social security disability," you would explain what to look for in the medical records for support of disability. You could tie the legal requirements of Social Security Disability (which you should know) to the medical information, but you wouldn't offer to explain the legal issues involved.

If you feel your writing skills need improvement, consider taking a course at your local college. No local college? Then buy a good book (or several) and study on your own. Ask a friend with good writing skills to help you. Don't trust thinking, "I think this is how you spell/punctuate/pluralize/etc. this."

> *...buy a good book (or several) and study on your own*

Always make sure by referring to your resources such AS THE CHICAGO MANUAL OF STYLE, THE GREGG REFERENCE MANUAL, Strunk and White's ELEMENTS OF STYLE, the AMERICAN HERITAGE DICTIONARY, WEBSTER'S DICTIONARY, TABER'S CYCLOPEDIC MEDICAL DICTIONARY, DORLAND'S MEDICAL DICTIONARY, etc., etc., etc. There is no excuse for not checking out your writing. Having good writing skill is necessary for doing your technical reports as well.

If you are interested in risk management at your hospital (or another hospital near you), offer to do a program for the staff there. That will show the risk management staff that you have the ability to do teaching/training. Programs that seem to go over well with hospital nurses include those that help them understand medical/nursing malpractice issues. You can also help nurses and staff develop good habits which could help

Good charting skills are always pertinent...

them avoid malpractice or at least mitigate litigation issues. Good charting skills are always pertinent since they can help protect you when you are involved in a lawsuit.

Another way to get involved in your own hospital's risk management department is to offer to help develop policy and procedure books. You might also offer to help prepare for an accreditation visit from JCAHO. You could learn a great deal just from being involved in this procedure.

PUBLIC RELATIONS TIPS

If you live in a small town, or a town that has a small newspaper, you can run a press release about your new business. Press releases are an announcement about your new business that SHOULD NOT SOUND LIKE AN ADVERTISEMENT. A press release is not an easy piece to write. You must provide enough interesting information for the piece to be like an informative story. Write clearly without using technical jargon or being too technical in your approach.

The upside of writing a press release is that most people are curious as to how nurses work with lawyers. It is also to your advantage that you are a local person and thus there is likely to be more interest. If you have completed schooling of some sort toward developing your LNC business, you can always send in the "news" of your completion of the course, and what your plans are in the future.

Sometimes, a paper is unwilling to run a press release or story about you unless you pay for an ad for your new business. This may be a small price to pay to get a story <u>and a picture of you</u>. The ad probably won't bring you any business, but it may be worth it to get a story written up about you.

The press release should be creative and <u>short</u>. It may be helpful

The press release should be creative and <u>short</u>

to go to the newspaper office and ask for help from someone there. Find out what they would be more likely to print. Also, provide them with a good photo. Ask them what they prefer in the way of photos. They may want a black and white print or they may prefer a slide. Be as helpful as possible in getting the story in the paper. The best case scenario might be that they become interested in what you do and offer to have one of their reporters do a story on you. That is even better than a press release–but you still need to do your homework or this will likely never happen to you.

Another possibility is if you to arrange to speak at the local bar association, you might ask to have that covered by the paper–

and have their photographer take the picture and their reporter write up the story. It helps to be able to tie in with events the paper is likely to cover anyway.

It may seem like a lot of trouble, but it does give you some credibility to be written about in the paper. Make sure you never tell any information about any of the cases in which you are involved. You never know who might personally be affected in your immediate area. Beside that fact, you have promised not to breach the confidentiality of your cases. Even taking the case out of context can be a slippery issue. If you must give a case example, find one that is written up from another source (such as a legal newspaper). You could use a case that you did in an entirely different locale (and is over with)–and still take it out of context so that no confidentiality will be breached. Although transcripts of court cases are available to the public, medical records should not be. Show your integrity with confidentiality. You are not the media.

ADVANCED—AND MORE COSTLY—MARKETING

There are other marketing strategies not covered in this guide. We purposely have not covered some of the more expensive types of marketing such as: Setting up a booth at large meetings; sending clients novelties such as calendars or pens or cups, etc.; running ads in legal papers, the Martindale-Hubbell Directory, the American Bar Association Directory, or other directories.

You can get your business well on its way without using these more expensive methods. However, as your business grows, you may want to consider some of those options. Our special report on advanced marketing methods can be ordered if you are interested in pursuing these.

The Bottom Line

☑ Be sure that pro bono work is not just work for free.

☑ Get to know your Legal Aid Society.

☑ Develop your speaking skills and apply them well.

☑ Learn to write well and use this skill in writing articles as well as your reports.

☑ Do a press release or try to get the newspaper interested in doing an article on you and your new career.

☑ Never breach confidentiality of the medical records.

People only see what they are prepared to see.
Ralph Waldo Emerson

SECTION 15 - ESTABLISHING YOUR CREDIBILITY

Establishing and maintaining your credibility requires that you constantly manage four elements: Your professional image, your work product, your dependability, and your ethics.

YOUR PROFESSIONAL IMAGE

Dress, if you think it doesn't matter, you may be "clueless"

Your image is important. It sends a subtle, but important, message about you. The first impression you make with your client should be your very best. In large part, this initial impression is made from your appearance and behavior; the impression is often made before you say anything. You will want to look and act like the professional you are. Indeed, you want to look like someone who should be charging the kind of hourly rates you will be charging.

...you want to look like someone who should be charging the kind of hourly rates you will be charging.

Occasionally, we come across an aspiring LNC who says, "Why should it matter what I wear? I have the knowledge, skills, and expertise that a client wants and needs. Why should they care about how I'm dressed?"

If this is your attitude, you are under suspicion of being clueless…

If this is your attitude, you are under suspicion of being clueless. And, in fact, there is a high probability that you will be unable to market your services as an LNC successfully.

How you dress is up to you. However, what it says about you is up to the person who is observing you. DRESS FOR SUCCESS guru, John Molloy, says if you think what you wear doesn't matter, consider this; go to your closet and put something on that doesn't make a statement about you. Even if you emerge totally naked, it will say something about you.

How you dress is up to you… what it says about you is up to the person who is observing you.

John Sez:
While we're on the topic of image here's another little rant.
I tell my graduate students that a good haircut can enhance your image significantly. This is particularly true for women. A good haircut is an investment in your image just as a well-made suit would be. Start noticing women's hair as you watch TV or visit professional offices. Notice the difference between those who have a good haircut and the rest. We're talking $50 and up here for a good one.

If, after your initial visit, you observe a different style of dress in your client's office, you may want to make some adjustments. However, tee shirts, jeans, and sneakers, even if that's what they are wearing, may not be quite how you want to present yourself. Err on the side of overdressing.

> **Betty's comment:**
> Many firms have "casual Friday. " If you visit a firm on Friday, don't assume that
> is their normal mode of dress.

A great tip on dressing

When visiting a client's office, observe what the attorneys—male
and female-are wearing, particularly if you are female. This
should be your clue as to what is appropriate for you. You may
notice that the secretaries or non-attorney staff may be dressed
differently than the attorneys. Numerous books on professional
presentation suggest you dress to the level of the person <u>above</u>
you. In any case, you want to be considered as a professional so
dressing like other professionals in the firm is a must.

> **John Sez:**
> If your marketing call yields some future work, do not make the mistake of
> appearing at your next visit dressed radically different. It makes you seem
> manipulative. You must continue to maintain your professional image.

The current situation with dress in the legal world

Although it may sound antiquated or sexist, some conservative
law firms and <u>most courts</u> frown upon women wearing pants
suits (or any pants outfit). Until you are sure of the acceptance
of this form of professional dress, we recommend that you wear
a skirted suit or business-type dress. This holds for female
attorneys as well. Hey! These same people don't like men to
wear earrings or being without a tie either, so it isn't all one-
gender bias.

John's rules for dress and appearance

❑ A black or navy blue business suit with a white blouse or shirt is always appropriate for your first meeting.

❑ For men, the minimum is a blazer and tie. Ties with pictures of your dog, your truck, or a popular brand of beer may not set the right tone.

❑ Cocktail dresses are seldom appropriate—especially when worn with feather boas.

❑ Closed shoes are highly recommended—but that doesn't mean Nikes, Reeboks, or Doc Martins.

❑ Monitor your jewelry; if you have been struck by lightning on more than one occasion, you may be wearing too much.

❑ Pearls with a tube top may be understated elegance but never when meeting with clients and never before April.

❑ When within 100 miles or less of a client, never, ever chew gum.

❑ Be aware of nervous habits—don't swing your foot or twirl your hair.

❑ A professional leather folio/note pad holder is an excellent accessory, since you will want to be taking notes while meeting with your client. Borrowing your child's Star Wars notebook doesn't have the same cachet.

❑ A decent pen may not enhance your image, but a 29 cent pen sure can detract from it.

YOUR WORK PRODUCT

> **John Sez:**
> This section is a continuation of our discussion about your professional image. It all fits together to make one big package. Quality clothing, accessories, haircut, note folio, pen, and now the quality of your work product.

The quality of your work product says volumes about you and your professionalism. The quality of your work begins with your written output. Misspelled words, poor grammar, and typos send the wrong message and can quickly

Misspelled words, poor grammar, and typos send the wrong message...

erode confidence in your work. It suggests that if you don't care enough to present clean, clear, correct copy, then you may not be concerned about the content either.

You must get in the habit of running your grammar and spell checker frequently. However, be aware that the spell checker does not correct all errors, and, while the grammar checker is a help, it also offers some erroneous data. You MUST edit the copy with

You MUST edit your copy with and eagle eye....

an eagle eye yourself—watching for typos, punctuation correctness, spelling, grammar, as well as content clarity. This is best done at least a day after the work has been completed, to give time between the preparation and the editing.

> **Betty's Comments:**
> If you find errors in the printed copy before you send it out, correct them and print out another copy. White-out and handwritten corrections are not only tacky but also unprofessional.

The quality of paper and envelopes used by you also influences the perception of your image. Make sure your materials are as professional looking as you.

You should be using professional level word-processing software that has excellent spelling and grammar checkers built in. You must also seriously consider purchasing a laser printer. The quality is far superior to all of the less expensive dot matrix, ink jet, and color ink jet printers on the market. All the law firms we are familiar with use laser printers as their main output device. You want your output to look as professional as your client's does.

If you are using a word-processing service or a secretary, make certain you review carefully all output from them. They may be unfamiliar with medical terms in particular. Additionally, you need to ascertain that their grammar is correct. Besides that, you need to assure yourself that the content as YOU dictated it is clear, well-organized, and grammatically correct.

John Sez:
Here's a tip on software. The latest figures show that 70% of the US market is using a Microsoft product as their main program. This is usually Microsoft Word or the Office 97 (or Office 2000) package. 14% of the market uses WordPerfect. The remaining 16% use a potpourri of programs. Based purely on the numbers I recommend Microsoft Word. (Like Bill Gates needs another buck!) (However, Betty insists that many law firms use WordPerfect—and WordPerfect is her favorite. Whatever you use, make it a first rate word-processing program.)

DEPENDABILITY

One of the quickest ways we know to wreck your carefully cultivated image is to develop a reputation for not being dependable. Your reputation can suffer serious damage from your inability or unwillingness to be dependable. Examples of not being dependable include not delivering work product as

Your reputation can suffer serious damage from your inability or unwillingness to be dependable

promised; being unwilling or unable to provide services when requested; promising more than you can deliver; not following up as promised; not returning calls promptly. The AALNC Code of Ethics and Conduct (see "Ethics" below) speaks in terms of being "accountable for responsibilities accepted and actions performed." So, there you have it. You are not only considered undependable but unethical.

A client may equate your lack of dependability in any one of the issues above as indicating you can't be counted on for other pertinent issues—such as confidentiality or thorough research. Remember, trust is a major factor in this relationship. When a client knows he can depend on you, he is much more willing to turn over a complex project to you.

> **Betty's comment:**
> In a home-office-based business, having members of the family take calls and forgetting to give you the message doesn't excuse you in the eyes of your clients. You need to be business-like if you plan to have a business.

ETHICS

American Bar Association Ethics

Despite the many jokes that circulate about the legal profession and lawyers, ethics are of great concern to them. The vast majority of people in the legal industry conduct themselves in an honest and ethical manner. Trust is a cornerstone on which you build client relations.

As a person working in this industry, you are expected to KNOW the requirements of legal ethics as well as follow them.

You should be at least familiar with the American Bar Association's Canons of Ethics for attorneys. A thorough review of the Model Rules and Codes for attorneys, as set out by the ABA, can be found in their publication, *ABA Compendium of Professional Responsibility – Rules and Standards.*

The ethical issues are sometimes specific attorney issues—such as they may not share contingency fees with non-lawyers. The work product you provide falls under the contingency fee category. Another reason you should never work on a contingency basis is that it is unethical for the lawyer to even ask this.

Your ethics are very important.

Examples of ethical issues are:

❏   You must tell your clients the bad news as well as the good. They are paying you to provide them with the medical facts and clarification related to those facts.

❏   Inflated billing for any reason is a breach of ethics. (Charging for time spent learning how to do normal LNC work should not be billed.)

❏   Do not misrepresent yourself to the lawyer concerning your experience or education—either clinical nursing or legal nurse consulting.

❏   Always be aware of conflicts of interest of whatever cause and inform the client of these.

❏   And last—do not even give the appearance of trying to practice law if you are not a lawyer. Some nurses seem to think they know the law better than the attorney. You are there to provide medical insight—not to run the case.

American Association of Legal Nurse Consultants Ethics

In the clinical areas, we are expected to have and follow a code of ethics in dealing with patients. Using our knowledge and skills in another facet of nursing does not diminish our ethical responsibilities—including respect for the client, confidentiality, and integrity.

The AALNC has developed a Code of Ethics and Conduct for the LNC with which you should be familiar. You can obtain a copy of this Code of Ethics and Conduct from the AALNC organization (see Section 1 for AALNC address). On the next page, we have summarized some aspects of the AALNC Code of Ethics.

John Sez:
This information is not a substitute for you actually reading these ethical codes. You need to get the full version from AALNC.

PROTECT YOUR CREDIBILITY

Once you have established your professional image and have shown yourself dependable, ethical, and a provider of quality work product, you must not let your image be tarnished. Don't take chances with attorneys, or even other LNCs, who tempt you to cross the line. If you don't have a good name, you'll have nothing.

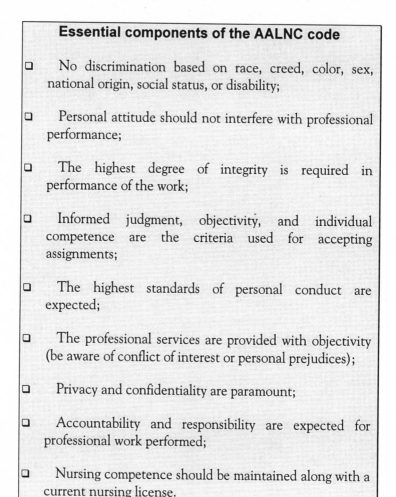

Essential components of the AALNC code

❑ No discrimination based on race, creed, color, sex, national origin, social status, or disability;

❑ Personal attitude should not interfere with professional performance;

❑ The highest degree of integrity is required in performance of the work;

❑ Informed judgment, objectivity, and individual competence are the criteria used for accepting assignments;

❑ The highest standards of personal conduct are expected;

❑ The professional services are provided with objectivity (be aware of conflict of interest or personal prejudices);

❑ Privacy and confidentiality are paramount;

❑ Accountability and responsibility are expected for professional work performed;

❑ Nursing competence should be maintained along with a current nursing license.

The Bottom Line

☑ Cultivate your professional image in a "dress for success" style.

☑ How you dress is up to you. However, recognize that others interpret the message through their perceptions.

☑ Your clear, correct, clean work product is part of your professional image and suggests the content was considered as carefully.

☑ Being dependable is, for your clients, an absolute necessity.

☑ Ethics are non-negotiable.

Notes

Remember, people will judge you by your actions,
not your intentions. You may have a heart of gold—but so does a
hard-boiled egg.
Anonymous

SECTION 16 - HOW TO KEEP CLIENTS ONCE YOU GET THEM

Getting new clients is a good thing; however, if you can't keep clients, your business will eventually suffer. This section points out some ways you can keep your name in front of clients as well as "keep them happy."

DO WHAT YOU HAVE BEEN DOING TO GET CLIENTS— ONLY EXPAND IT

In this guide, we have told you the important things about identifying prospects and making clients of those prospects. Much of that same information is applicable here. You must present yourself professionally, provide impeccable work product, keep your word, and have the highest integrity in all matters. This section repeats and emphasizes concepts you need to expand. They are presented as four rules for a good client relationship. These rules address implementing what we have already spoken about.

A Reality Check

It should be said up front, that you WILL lose some clients through no fault of your own. They may end up hiring a full-time LNC (and you may not wish to do that); they may lose their clients for whom they did the medical work; the firm may break up and re-form in a different manner. These are a few of the scenarios that may result in your losing a client. Try never to lose a client through your own fault, through poor work, or inappropriate billing, or unethical behavior, or …you know the drill.

FOUR RULES FOR A GOOD CLIENT RELATIONSHIP

Rule #1: Be sure you understand what is asked of you

The first item of importance about doing a case (after

> *…be very clear about what the client wants you to do.*

determining no conflict of interest) is to BE VERY CLEAR ABOUT WHAT THE CLIENT WANTS YOU TO DO. Many times you know more about what you can offer them than they know; however, they know the limit of the work they want you to do. For example, if Plaintiff Attorney, Esq. asks you to review a case for merit and report back to her, don't spend extensive time on the record paginating, binding, etc. just because you think there is merit, and they might want you to do it later. Even if you think there is merit to the case, they might decide not to take it—and that is their call, not yours. They did not ask you to spend—and BILL that much time and will resent paying it or will refuse to pay you for the time, because they did not ask for that work to be done. You should be aware that, most of the time, the actual plaintiff pays for pre-filing (before it is a lawsuit) work done by you—out of his pocket.

Betty's comment:
It is a good idea to have a "new file" or "new case" form or template to be sure you get all the information you need on a case. We have included a sample form in the Appendix B.
Also, don't forget to use your contract agreement to clarify the work that you are expected to do as well as the parameters of completion time and costs.

Rule #2: Do more than is required of you

If you are clear about what the attorney wants you to do—and it is a good idea to get that in writing through your contract (see appendix for form), provide a little something extra for that client, especially at the beginning of the relationship.

Provide some research article abstracts (that you can find by searching Medline or PubMed online) that relate to the issue in the case. Or do a quick time line of some specific and pertinent issue that would be useful in clarifying the issues of the case. The trick is to provide something extra to show the client more ways you can offer help in addition to just providing a summary or merit review of the medical records.

Please be clear that this is a freebie. Make sure the client understands you are not charging for this little something extra. When you write your cover letter for the summary/work product you do, clearly state that you have provided the client with "six abstracts regarding the issue at hand," or a "time line of the vital signs of the evening that is being litigated"—or whatever you have provided. Be sure to include that, "There is no charge for this since you did not request it." Make a point that you can, and do, have additional means to be of value in the client's cases.

> **Betty's comment:**
> Also, when you bill the client, itemize what you did that was extra and put "no charge" or n/c.

Once that client is familiar with what you have to offer, you may still want to send additional, <u>free,</u> items. An example of this would be to send an abstract, or the article itself, which relates to an issue of a case you have recently summarized for them. The point is that you had them on your mind when you read about the issue that they are litigating. Although you may have completed and sent the client the work product they requested, you still kept them in mind and found an article pertinent to their case. Like a marriage, you are showing you are not taking them for granted and that you value the relationship. It is also a method of keeping your name current in their mind.

Rule #3: Keep informed by reading broadly

Following up on concepts above, you will have to keep informed about medical and nursing issues in order to be aware of articles that apply to your clients' cases. There is so much information available on the Internet that it is easy to keep updated. Well, there is <u>so</u> much available that it may not be <u>easy,</u> but it certainly is accessible. You should make use of all that information and make it a point to read about the issues of some of the cases in which you have become involved.

In addition to medical information, it is helpful to you to stay up with what is happening in the legal field. There are many sites on the Internet that present that information as well. If your city or community has a legal paper, you may find that of interest. To use a trite saying, "you are not an island" and keeping up with what is going on in the medical-legal world is of some importance to you.

Betty's comment:
However, don't believe everything you read—even in medical journals. Assess the information before you pass it on. Is it "peer reviewed?" Is it "good science?" Is it biased or prejudiced? What kind of research is it? Is it anecdotal or actual research and measurement? How many subjects were in the study? Also, don't suggest to the client that this study alone can win his case. It usually takes many studies combined to present a good case.

Rule #4: Follow up on your marketing

Keep the relationship fresh; continue to use your marketing skills on them. In addition to providing helpful (free) articles or abstracts, etc., it is also just good sense to follow up with your client and ask if they are satisfied with your work product. Ask what you can do to help them more. This kind of "check-up" can help you hone your skills as well as keeps your name in the minds of your clients.

Sometimes they will make truly valuable suggestions for improvement in your work product. Some will just prefer a certain way of doing reports. It is your responsibility to keep your client satisfied—not by always agreeing with them on a case, but by providing clear, well-documented, factual information about the case issues. And in a format that is creative and helpful. You are well on your way to being a successful LNC when you can do this.

The Bottom Line

☑ Do the basics: excellent work product, dependability, integrity, keep your promises.

☑ Bill your time appropriately and with specificity.

☑ Be professional—in appearance and in behavior.

☑ Send thank-you notes immediately.

☑ Return calls promptly.

☑ Know what the client wants from you—specifically.

☑ Do more than is required.

☑ Keep yourself informed and updated

☑ Be aware of, and avoid, potentially unethical issues.

☑ Ask how you can improve.

APPENDIX A – MARKETING CHECKLIST AND MARKETING FLOW SHEET

Contents:
Marketing Checklist
Marketing Flow Sheet

Marketing Check List

If you are going into business as an independent legal nurse consultant, you should review the items below to check your readiness for getting your business underway.

I. Complete a course in legal nurse consulting by one of the following methods:

- ☐ Self-study using appropriate materials
- ☐ Home study course
- ☐ Personal coach preparation
- ☐ Classroom course specifically designed for LNCs

II. Plan for the following legal requirements:

A. The legal form of your business
- ☐ Sole Proprietor
- ☐ Partnership*
- ☐ Subchapter S Corporation*

  *You will need an Attorney to help you set this up

B. State and local legal requirements:
- ☐ Business license requirements
- ☐ Zoning requirements (in the case of a home office)
- ☐ Subdivision restrictions on home based business
- ☐ Tax requirements involved in the legal form you elected

III. Assess your preparedness and personality in comparison to the following characteristics of successful LNCs:

- ☐ I am internally driven and a self-starter.
- ☐ I have objectively considered the requirements of having my own business.
- ☐ I have included my family in the planning and discussed the impact this will have on them.
- ☐ I have the perseverance to follow through on plans, promises, and problems.
- ☐ I am prepared for the valleys and peaks of billable work/cash flow.

☐ I have sufficient time and energy to put into a new business venture.

☐ I have the self-confidence and positive mental attitude necessary to accept responsibility and to handle problems that are likely to arise.

☐ I am willing to put the effort into marketing that it will take to become a successful LNC.

☐ I have a realistic concept of all that is required to run my office, market myself, develop a budget, manage my income and expenses, and provide the best possible work product for my clients.

☐ I am able to cope with problems with equanimity.

☐ I have the emotional stability to face the risks involved in owning my own business.

☐ I am willing to invest the time it takes to keep myself informed on current medical/nursing issues as well as those in the case I am currently preparing.

☐ I understand the need to keep up continuing education in nursing as well as in medical-legal issues.

☐ I have sufficient funds for my business start-up needs.

☐ I am able to assess my strengths and weaknesses in relation to my new business.

☐ I am able to take criticism from my clients and, in fact, understand that I should seek suggestions for improvement according to my clients needs.

IV. Develop a plan for your business[1]:

☐ Determine where your office will be located. (Be very specific, i.e. state exactly WHERE in your home.):

---

[1] Note that we purposely do not use "Business Plan." That term is appropriate when you are developing a business plan to present to banks, etc. to obtain money. However, we think you must have a PLAN for your business so that you know where you are going.

☐ Determine what computer/telephone/fax/printer hardware you have and what you will need to get your business up and running.

☐ Assess your computer software and determine if it is capable of providing high quality work product.

☐ Prepare a budget for any necessary equipment, supplies, filing needs, office support (if any help is planned), medical and nursing references for your office, and marketing, as well as for the ongoing upkeep of the office for at least one year.

☐ Develop a schedule of fees and hourly rates and a standard process for contracting work and billing hours.

☐ Plan printed materials, business cards, brochures, stationery, etc. with quality in mind.

☐ Orient the content of marketing materials towards solving client's problems.

☐ Understand the need for continuing marketing and develop a long term plan for such.

☐ Research potential clients and prepare to market them with specificity.

☐ Recognize the power of networking and have plans to or have begun developing your networks.

☐ Develop awareness of the organization(s) which offer support, education, and information for LNCs and have a plan to join such.

☐ Recognize the importance of keeping up with nursing and medical areas as well as the legal arena and plan to continue to study and develop your knowledge in these.

☐ Have good communication skills, both written and oral, that it takes to market myself appropriately and to provide a good work product for clients.

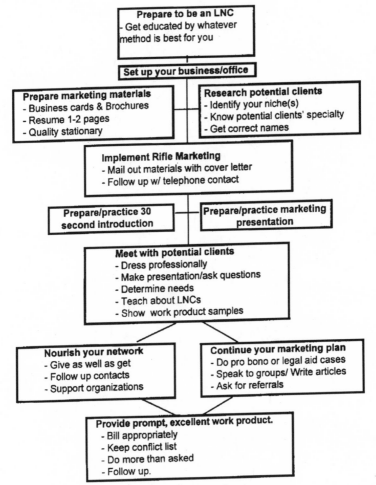

Prepare to be an LNC
- Get educated by whatever method is best for you

Set up your business/office

Prepare marketing materials
- Business cards & Brochures
- Resume 1-2 pages
- Quality stationary

Research potential clients
- Identify your niche(s)
- Know potential clients' specialty
- Get correct names

Implement Rifle Marketing
- Mail out materials with cover letter
- Follow up w/ telephone contact

Prepare/practice 30 second introduction

Prepare/practice marketing presentation

Meet with potential clients
- Dress professionally
- Make presentation/ask questions
- Determine needs
- Teach about LNCs
- Show work product samples

Nourish your network
- Give as well as get
- Follow up contacts
- Support organizations

Continue your marketing plan
- Do pro bono or legal aid cases
- Speak to groups/ Write articles
- Ask for referrals

Provide prompt, excellent work product.
- Bill appropriately
- Keep conflict list
- Do more than asked
- Follow up.

Marketing flow chart

Notes

APPENDIX B - BROCHURES, LETTERS, FORMS, ETC

Contents:
Sample brochure
Four sample letters
Two sample retainer forms
Client contact form
New File/Case Form

Brochures

The next two pages are an example of a brochure.

Paper stock: This is a Paper Direct, three color, and three-panel 38lb scored brochure. The main color is a light green, the heavy lines are either cranberry or black.

Panel 1: Notice the *Professional Medical Expertise* statement. This is a "benefit" statement.

Panel 2: Contains "benefit" statements, along with Betty's contact information.

Panel 3: If you have clients, it is good to list them. This helps legitimize you as a bona-fide LNC. If you're just starting out, put benefit statements in this panel until you start to get clients.

Panel 4: This panel is a teaching piece. It helps the Attorney understand what an LNC does.

Panel 5: This is a combination teaching/benefit piece. Notice that each statement starts with an action verb.

Panel 6: Betty's credibility is established with this panel. Notice that most of what is cited is relevant to attorneys.

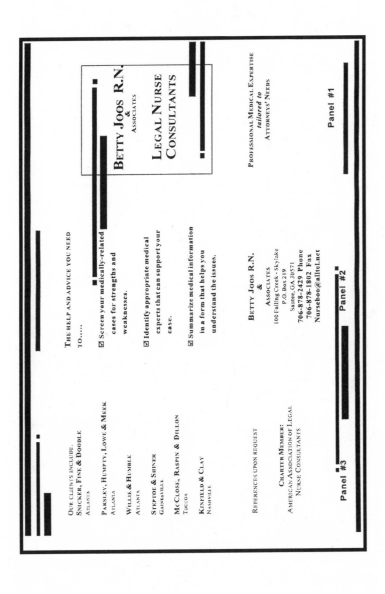

THE LEGAL NURSE CONSULTANT AS A MEMBER OF THE LITIGATION TEAM

Legal nurse consultants are registered nurses who have chosen to use their knowledge and expertise to help attorneys de-mystify the medical issues in legal cases. LNCs are involved in both plaintiff and defense cases.

As professionals, they follow their medical ethics of confidentiality in client communications as well as the ABA ethics.

Any case with medical issues involved offers a potential morass of information. The nurse consultant provides an insider's perspective on the practices and procedures of the healthcare industry as well as an in-depth understanding of the medical facts and patient care issues.

The LNC's work is time-saving and cost-effective in the litigation process and can provide the critical advantage you need to win your case.

A few brief examples:

An LNC noticed that a congenital spinal defect was documented on a previously unnoticed supplement to a radiologist's report. Testimony revealed that the congenital defect was the true cause of the litigant's problem rather than a slip and fall which had been the basis of the suit. *Result: the case settled for $800,000 less than the demand.*

Records not previously obtained from an evaluating neurologist held the key to the plaintiff's case. *Result: the Plaintiff's attorney settled the case for $300,000 more than had first been offered in settlement.*

Panel #4

OUR SERVICES

☐ Inform you regarding the medical facts and issues

☐ **Research** the literature regarding the medical issues

☐ **Review, organize, and analyze** medical records

☐ **Assess medically related damages** in personal injury cases or product liability cases

☐ Provide an **analysis** of a person's past medical history and it's relevance to the case at hand

☐ **Identify standards of care, causation, and damages** in medical malpractice cases

☐ **Prepare written summaries and reports,** of medical records, research findings, expert witness information (Provided on computer disk and/or paper)

☐ **Provide support in medical depositions**

☐ **Identify and obtain appropriate medical experts**

☐ Aid in preparing **demonstrative evidence and exhibits**

☐ **Collaborate in developing strategies for** medically related cases

☐ **Digest** medical depositions

Panel #5

BETTY JOOS, R.N., B.S.N., M.ED.

Betty Joos is an experienced legal nurse consultant. Her expertise in this field developed through a broad base of teaching, clinical nursing experience, as an honors graduate of the National Center for Paralegal Training in Atlanta, and by 12 years as a practicing legal nurse consultant.

Prior to legal nurse consulting, Betty was a college nursing instructor for over 15 years. Her clinical experience includes pediatrics, medical-surgical nursing, and emergency department nursing. She is a former Paramedic and director of an emergency medical training program. The melding of this broad experience and education with her paralegal training equips Betty with a unique ability to provide support for attorneys involved in cases with medical-legal issues.

Betty developed her LNC practice in Atlanta, starting as an in-house consultant with a firm that she kept as a major client after she became an independent practitioner.

Betty possesses excellent writing and literature research skills. She has published in the *American Journal of Nursing* and *Network: Journal for the Legal Nurse Consultant.* She helped develop, and teaches in, a program for Legal Nurse Consultants in Atlanta. As a professional in her own field, Betty will collaborate with you to develop a cost effective and winning approach to the medical issues involved in your case.

Panel #6

Betty Joos RN & Associates

100 Falling Creek
P O Box 219 ● Sautee, GA 30571 ● (706) 878-2429 ● Fax: (706) 878-1802

May 1, 2000

If your letter gets long such as this, you may need to decrease the font size to 11 point Times Roman or use a different font (as done here) such as Agaramond. You will have various letterhead choices–from your word processing programs–but may have to remove a space or two in the upper part of the letter to keep it to one page. But DO keep it to ONE PAGE.

Henry P. Gotcha, Esq.
Gotcha, Getcha, & Payme, P. A.
5000 Anywhere Street
P. 0. Box 5000
Everywhere, New State 0000 1

Dear Mr. Gotcha:

If you get a headache just looking at a large stack of medical records, let me tell you how using a legal nurse consultant can help relieve your headache by increasing your efficiency when preparing your next medically related case.

Legal nurse consultants are registered nurses with broad medical experience who provide you with the tools you need to make your medically related cases more winnable. Here is a brief sample of some of the things Betty Joos, RN & Associates do to help our clients be more successful:

> Our organization and analysis of medical records helps you quickly and efficiently pull together the issues in your case. Our clients tell us this is one of the biggest time-savers we provide.

> We research and provide the appropriate medical literature or standards of care for the medical issues to support your case in depositions or trial.

> We determine the type medical experts that you need to strengthen your case and help you locate the most appropriate expert.

> We can improve your understanding of the subtleties and nuances of the medical facts as well as offering insight into the working of hospitals, clinics, and other medical facilities to help you develop winning case strategies.

The enclosed brochure lists the services that we offer to our clients. I will call you shortly after you have received this letter to set up a 15 –20 minute meeting. The purpose of the meeting is threefold: (1) to get to meet you, (2) to learn more about your firm and the types of medically related problems you are encountering, and (3) to show you some examples of some of the ways we help our clients develop stronger cases.

I look forward to meeting you.

Sincerely,

Betty Joos, R.N., B.S.N., M.Ed.
Legal Nurse Consultant

Betty Joos, RN & Associates

Betty Joos, RN BSN MEd
P O Box 219
100 Falling Creek
Sautee, Georgia 30571
(706) 878-2429
Fax: (706) 878-1802

May 1, 2000

Henry P. Gotcha, Esq.
Gotcha, Getcha, & Payme, P. A.
5000 Anywhere Street
P. O. Bo 5000
Everywhere, New State   00001

> Note this is a plaintiff-oriented letter.
> The font in this letter in size 12 Times
> New Roman– a commonly used font
> in professional circles.

Dear Mr. Gotcha:

Since plaintiff medical malpractice cases are among your specialities, I would like to show you how using a legal nurse consultant can increase your efficiency and improve you chances of a better outcome in your cases.

Legal nurse consultants are nurses with broad medical experience who can provide you with the tools to make your medical malpractice cases more winnable. This begins with assessing the merit of the numerous medical malpractice allegations brought to your firm. Determining merit on the issues can help you prevent loss of valuable time and money. In meritorious cases, medical records can be organized and summarized to your preference. Written reports can be prepared in narrative form, chronological format, or issue time lines. On-point medical literature research and text resources can be provided by way of abstracts or full articles which can be used to support your medical issues in deposition or trial. Appropriate medical experts can be identified and located to make your case presentation stronger. A nurse consultant offers insight into the working of hospitals, clinics, and other medical facilities, as well as explaining medical terms and their connections in your specific case.

The enclosed brochure lists the services we can offer to help you in your work. I will call you shortly after you have received this letter to set up a 15 to 20 minute meeting for further discussion of the services and resources we provide. Thank you for your time and consideration.

Sincerely,

Betty Joos, RN & Associates
Legal Nurse Consultants

Betty Joos, RN & Associates
100 Falling Creek
P O Box 219
Sautee, GA 30571
(706) 878-2429Fax:
(706) 878-1802

May 1, 2000

Henry P. Gotcha, Esq.
Gotcha, Getcha, & Payme, P. A.
5000 Anywhere Street
P. 0. Box 5000
Everywhere, New State 0000 1

> Note in this letter that we have used
> **BOLD** to highlight specific value-
> added aspects of LNCs' work. the font
> is 12 pt. Times New Roman.

Dear Mr. Gotcha:

If you get a headache just looking at a large stack of medical records, let me tell you how using a
legal nurse consultant can **increase your efficiency and improve case outcomes** in your
medically related cases.

Legal nurse consultants are registered nurses with broad medical experience who provide you
with the tools you need to **make your medically related cases more winnable.** Our clients tell
us that the organization and analysis of medical records is one of the biggest **time-savers** we
provide. We offer written reports in narrative form, chronological format, or time lines of
medical issues. Because we have medical expertise, we frequently uncover issues and facts that
are easily overlooked by non-medical persons. Legal nurse consultants have the advantage of
insight into the working of hospitals, clinics, and other medical facilities. In many cases,
**winning or losing a case is often dependent on your understanding of the subtleties and
nuances of the medical politics as well as facts.**

The enclosed brochure lists the numerous services that we can provide to our clients. I will call
you shortly after you have received this letter to set up a 15 to 20 minute meeting. The purpose of
the meeting is threefold: (1) to get to meet you, (2) to learn more about your firm and the types of
medically related problems you are encountering, and (3) to show you some examples of some of
the ways we help our clients develop stronger cases.

I look forward to talking with you.

Sincerely,

Betty Joos, R.N., B.S.N., M.Ed.
Legal Nurse Consultant

BETTY JOOS RN & ASSOCIATES

100 FALLING CREEK
P O BOX 219 • SAUTEE, GA 30571 • (706) 878-2429 • FAX: (706) 878-1802

May 1, 2000

Abigail Holdem
Attorney-at-law
Holdem, Holdem, & Winnum
1000 Near Your Place
Anywhere, Your State 00010

Note that this letter is <u>defendant oriented</u> and is done in
BernhardMod BT font in 12 point size [*this note is done
in Times Roman–11 pt*]. The templates [*forms*] for the
letterhead in your word processing programs come with
their own font variation–some you may like and some
not. Keeping your style of letterhead–and font--
consistent looks more professional than trying to be
different each time you correspond with a client.

Dear Ms. Holdem:

Defending medical malpractice suits is a challenging business. Sometimes the difference in
winning a case is dependant on your understanding of the subtleties and nuances of the medical
issues involved. As a legal nurse consultant with over 20 years of clinical experience and more
than a decade of medical-legal consulting experience, I would like to show you how Betty Joos,
RN & Associates can help you handle your cases more efficiently and develop case strategies that
improve case outcomes.

One of the biggest time-savers we provide in our behind-the-scenes service, is the essential
organization and analysis of the medical records, provided to you in a format of your choosing – a
chronological summation, a narrative report, or a time-line of the issues. Medical literature
research is offered to support your strategy of the case and appropriate experts can be determined
and located. Knowledge gained through clinical experience offers you insight into the workings of
hospitals, clinics, and doctors' offices, giving you an advantage of understanding some the
"political" issues of a medical practice as well..

The enclosed brochure describes the services offered to our clients. I will call you shortly after
you receive this letter to set up a 15 minute meeting at your convenience. The purposes of the
meeting are to learn more about the types of medically-related problems you are encountering as
well as to show you some examples of the ways we help our clients develop stronger cases. I look
forward to talking with you.

Sincerely,

Betty Joos, RN, BSN, MEd
Legal Nurse Consultant

SAMPLE FORM– Use what is helpful
****
RETAINER AGREEMENT

Date

Law firm
Address
Project: [give the plaintiff's name or the case name if possible]
Requested by: [name attorney]

I hereby retain [*your name*] as a Legal Nurse Consultant to provide review and summary of medical records in this instant case....research of the medical literature....[*whatever the client has requested you do. BE AS EXPLICIT AS YOU CAN IN RE WHAT HAS BEEN REQUESTED OF YOU. If you were asked to organize and paginate, etc. be sure to put that in. ALSO BE CLEAR AS TO WHETHER YOU ARE ACTING AS A NURSE EXPERT OR A BEHIND-THE-SCENES CONSULTANT. This can save a great deal of grief if at some later time if you are asked to be an expert. As an expert, you would charge more per hour, and your work becomes discoverable. For example, if this is behind-the-scenes work you might say:*]
It is understood that [*your name*] is not the nurse expert for this case, but is providing work product which is not discoverable.

I agree to pay to [*your name*], Legal Nurse Consultant [*or nurse expert*], the hourly fee of [*state your dollar amount fee*] for all work performed on this instant case, plus any out-of-pocket expenses incurred, including but not limited to, photocopies, shipping/postage, toll calls, travel expenses, research costs. I understand I will be billed [*monthly if you think the project will go beyond one month, or at the completion of the project if it is a one-time request*]. I also agree to provide a retainer of [*$$ amount – estimate about how many hours you think it might take and ask for about 50% or more of that amount*] at the outset, along with the first documents sent.

Ms./Mr. [*your name*] has advised me that she maintains a conflict-of-interest check on the files she is involved with, and will notify me if a conflict situation arises or is known of at this time. It is also confirmed that Ms./Mr. [*your name*] understands that confidentiality of all the documents in this case is primary, and that she agrees not to divulge any confidential information which she may become privy to while working on this instant case.

I agree the above terms set out the parameters of the work requested in this case, and my signature is confirmation of acceptance of such terms.

                            _____
                            [Attorney name]

                            _____
                            [LNC's name]

SAMPLE FORM EXAMPLE
●●●
RETAINER AGREEMENT

Date: February 11, 1999

Pink, Purple & Powerful
123 Find Us Road
Anywhere, Georgia 00000

Project: Friction v. Fraction, M. D., et al.
Requested by: Susan Foundgold, Esq.

I hereby retain Betty Joos as a Legal Nurse Consultant to provide review and summary of medical records in this instant case. Organization, pagination, and binding of all medical records are requested along with a chronological summary of all currently provided records. Medical literature research on the issues involved is also requested. However, only abstracts are desired, not library retrieval of articles, at the present time. These items are as we discussed in our phone conversation on February 10, 2000. It is understood that Ms. Joos is not the nurse expert for this case, but is providing work product which is not discoverable.

I agree to pay to Ms. Joos, Legal Nurse Consultant, the hourly fee of $70 for all work performed on this instant case, plus any out-of-pocket expenses incurred, including but not limited to, photocopies, shipping/postage, toll calls, travel expenses, research costs. I understand I will be billed when the report and bound records are returned to my office. I also agree to provide a retainer of five hundred dollars [$500] at the outset, along with the first documents sent.

Ms. Joos has advised me that she maintains a conflict-of-interest check on the files she is involved with and will notify me if a conflict situation arises or is known of at this time. It is also confirmed that Ms. Joos understands that confidentiality of all the documents in this case is primary, and that she agrees not to divulge any confidential information which she may become privy to while working on this instant case.

I agree the above terms set out the parameters of the work requested in this case and my signature is confirmation of acceptance of such terms.

_____

Susan Foundgold, Esq.

_____

Betty Joos, RN, BSN, MEd

Copy 1

Client Contact Form

In Section 11, we talk about Meeting with Prospects. The Client Contact Form is designed to help you manage your marketing contacts with potential clients. Prepare this form for each potential client you contact.

TIP: Prepare a master copy of the form on your word processing program and save it as a template. Both Microsoft Word and Wordperfect can create custom templates, check your HELP menu for instructions. When you get ready to use the form all you have to do is open the template and start filling in the blanks.

PRE-INTERVIEW MARKETING: Use this section to document your marketing efforts.

CLIENT INTERVIEW INFORMATION: Fill in as much of the information as possible prior to your meeting. You should have already done your homework to obtain the information about the attorney and firm. You should also prepare specific questions for this potential client.

AT THE INTERVIEW: Refer to your form for the questions you have prepared and write your notes about the responses.
Don't forget to ask for their business and ask for other referrals.

AFTER THE INTERVIEW: Do this immediately after the interview. In your car, before you leave the parking lot, is a good place for this. Classify the potential client according to the hierarchy of prospects. Make progress notes about the interview.

POST MEETING FOLLOW-UP: Send a thank-you note (preferably handwritten) immediately (no later than the day after.) Plan for follow-up contacts (send appropriate articles, your newsletter, etc.) and keep track of each date and type of contact you make. Keep contact for at least six to eight months.

John Sez:
If you don't like our Client Contact form it's okay to design your own.

Client Contact Form

PRE-INTERVIEW MARKETING

Marketing Letter sent: (Date) _____   Meeting date: _____

Phone contact(s) (Dates)_____

Referred by: _____ (Permission to use name?) _____

Met at (or first contact if other than by letter) _____

****

CLIENT INTERVIEW INFORMATION

DATE/TIME interview scheduled: _____

FIRM NAME: _____

ATT'Y NAME: _____   # OF ATTORNEYS IN FIRM: _____

Address:_____   Phone: _____

_____   FAX: _____

E-mail: _____   Web site: _____

SECRETARY: _____ PARALEGAL/LEGAL ASSISTANT(S): _____

Personal Info about attorney from research: (such as PLAINTIFF or DEFENSE; school attended, etc.)

Specialties of attorney according to pre-interview research: (can find in Martindale Hubbell or sometimes at firm web site) – such as medical malpractice, personal injury, products liability...

Specialty according to atty's interview statements: (if any changes noted)

****

AT THE INTERVIEW

QUESTIONS: *(sample questions are given here – you should develop your own according to need and leave space for responses. Don't forget, you may have to help the attorney understand what LNCs do.)*

- ☐ What are your greatest problems in medical cases?
- ☐ Who usually does your medical reviews and summaries?
- ☐ Have you ever used a nurse consultant before?
- ☐ What did you find helpful in using an LNC? (Or not helpful–so you can continue to categorize this potential client.)
- ☐ What cases do you have now that might use the expertise of an LNC?

ANTICIPATED PROBLEMS WITH WHICH I CAN HELP: (Circle during or after interview)

Organization of records   Standards of Care   Merit Reviews (if Plaintiff)

Medical lit research   Identify Experts   Locate experts

TIP: Don't forget to ask for their business and referrals.
****

AFTER THE INTERVIEW

CLASSIFICATION OF THE POTENTIAL CLIENT (circle)
HOT   AWARE BUT NO CASE   AWARE BUT UNCONVINCED   UNAWARE

Other problems identified by client during interview:

Progress notes about the interview:

****

POST-MEETING FOLLOW-UP

THANK YOU NOTE SENT (date): _____

OTHER CONTACTS
    1.
    2.
    Etc. through at least six to eight months of contacts.
ADDITIONAL FOLLOW-UP:

INFORMATION FOR
NEW FILE/CASE FORM

Referring attorney:_____ P or D

Address:_____

Phone:_____ FAX:_____

Contact person:_____

Case Name:_____ Case No._____

Type of Case: Personal injury _____   Medical Malpractice _____
          Product liability _____   Other (E.g., review for merit)_____

Date filed:_____ (Or Statute of Limitations)

Court:_____

Discovery ends:_____

Plaintiff's name(s):_____

Date of birth: _____ SS#:_____

Date of incident:_____

Description of incident:

Plaintiff's allegations:

Name of opposing attorney(s): _____

 Phone No.:_____   Contact name:_____

Conflict of interest checked?:   _____

Case Name:_____

Client name:_____

Work requested by attorney-client: Review for Merit   NO report

Organize records   Paginate   Bind records

  Summarize   Time line   Narrative   Deposition
                                                      questions

Determine expert   Locate expert   Contact expert

Research expert's credentials/publications   Literature research   Literature
                                                                        report

Other _____

Medical records: (List below records which are received already and those which
you have requested that the law firm get in addition or which they have already
requested and plan to send later. Include the name of the facility and the physicians
of that facility as well as the dates the records were received by you. Use as many
pages as needed for this.)

(R) received; (N) needed; (R-N) requested, not received; (NR) Not requested yet

Notes

APPENDIX C - REFERENCES AND RESOURCES

REFERENCES AND RESOURCES

WEB SITES:

There are many web sites that are useful to the LNC. However, in this section we only include those that are helpful in your marketing preparation and implementation. There are bound to be web sites we have overlooked; you can let us know ones that have been helpful to you by checking our own web site, sky-lake.com and sending us an e-mail. We will include these in our update for the marketing guide.

http://www.aalnc.org	American Association of Legal Nurse Consultants	Excellent networking group; good for continuing update on LNC information; poor link responses
http://www.abanet.org	American Bar Association	Good for networking; can join and receive excellent resources; can search in Public section for lawyers (but not the best method)
http://www.ambest.com /legal/atsearch.html	A.M. Best 's Directory of Recommended Insurance Attorneys and Adjusters	Good resource for locating defense attorneys in specific cities; information provided is not as complete as Martindale-Hubbell

http://www.atlanet.org	Association of Trial Lawyers of America	Plaintiff lawyer's association; can join ATLA, otherwise, much of the web site is off limits; can search to locate ATLA attorney members via "Public"
http://www.dogpile.com	Dogpile search engine	A multi-search engine that "fetches" information from a number of excellent sources. I have not had problems with getting porno on this search engine.
http://hg.org/	Hieros Gamos (Greek—means harmonization of seeming opposites)	Good overall resource for legal information; lists bar associations
http://ins.lawnt.com/	Law Net	Another good resource for locating defense attorneys specifically.
http://lawnewsnetwork.com	Law News Network	Good general update of legal news; can locate stories about attorneys in your area at times.
http://lawoffice.com	West Legal Directory online	Can search for attorneys online via Find a Lawyer (select professional malpractice and area you want)
http://martindalehubbell.com	Martindale Hubbell Law Directory	The best resource, in my opinion; can get more specific information on attorneys
http://sba.gov/	Small Business Association online	Lots of help for starting up your business

ASSOCIATIONS:

American Association of Legal Nurse Consultants
4700 W. Lake Avenue, Glenview IL 60025
877/402-2562
(Request the Practice Standards and Ethics booklets from AALNC)

American Bar Association
750 North Lake Shore Drive, Chicago IL 60611
800/285-2221

Association of Trial Lawyers of America
1050 31ˢᵗ Street NW, Washington DC 20007
800/424-2725

BOOKS:

ABA COMPENDIUM OF PROFESSIONAL RESPONSIBILITY RULES AND STANDARDS. American Bar Association: Chicago, 1997.

Covey, Stephen R. THE 7 HABITS OF HIGHLY EFFECTIVE PEOPLE. Simon & Schuster, Inc.: New York, 1990.

Davidson, Jeff. THE COMPLETE IDIOT'S GUIDE TO MANAGING YOUR TIME. Alpha Books, A Pearson Education Macmillan Company: Indianapolis, IN, 1995.

Glaser, Connie Brown and Barbara Steinberg Smalley. MORE POWER TO YOU! HOW WOMEN CAN COMMUNICATE THEIR WAY TO SUCCESS. Warner Books: New York, 1992.

Lavington, Camille with Stephanie Losee. YOU'VE ONLY GOT THREE SECONDS: HOW TO MAKE THE RIGHT IMPRESSION IN YOUR BUSINESS AND SOCIAL LIFE. Doubleday: New York, 1997.

Roane, Susan. HOW TO WORK A ROOM: A GUIDE TO SUCCESSFULLY MANAGING THE MINGLING. Shapolsky Publishers, Inc.: New York, 1988.

INDEX

Notes